ADVANCE PRAISE FOR

JUST BREATHE

"This is a timely and essential book for our challenged world. Dan Brulé is a true master and deeply inspiring. *Just Breathe* is free medicine that will not only bring you optimal health, but also expand your consciousness."

—Mark Divine, retired Navy SEAL, founder/CEO of SEALfit and *New York Times* bestselling author of *The Way of the SEAL* and *Unbeatable Mind*

"Dan Brulé's new book is a fascinating and practical guide to the overlooked importance of the breath for creativity, vitality, and healing."

—BARNET BAIN, author of *The Book of Doing and Being* and producer of *What Dreams May Come*

"Excellent content and presentation. I will be very happy when more of my students and associates contribute as much as Dan has to the enlightenment and evolution of humanity through breathwork."

—LEONARD ORR, founder of Rebirth International

"Dan Brulé weaves together breathing physiology, psychology, and spirituality in uniquely practical ways that most anyone can learn for improving health and performance. His writing style is crisp, clear, personal, easy to read, and even exciting. His book is a 'must read' not only for breathworkers, healthcare practitioners, and yoga-meditation fans, but also for virtually anyone who suspects that breathing might just be something important in their lives!"

—PETER M. LITCHFIELD, PhD, President of the Graduate School of Behavioral Health Sciences

"I love the way Dan gently enters breath mastery through awareness, relaxation, and breathing. His 'Wake Up!' 'Let Go!' and 'Take Charge' are the basics of what we all teach, but here in *Just Breathe* it is so clear and straightforward."

—DR. DAVID O'HARE, MD, author of *Heart Coherence 365*

"This book, which embodies Dan's life work, draws us in, inhales us into a fresh new state of awareness, of seeing how, even in the small moments of each day, we can transform our experiences with conscious breathing. Then it breathes us out into the world with freedom from habits and limitations, with wisdom from ancient traditions and modern science, and with the knowledge that it is quite possible to heal ourselves and others using the power of our breath."

—PATRICIA GERBARG, MD, Assistant Clinical Professor of Psychiatry, New York Medical College and coauthor of *The Healing Power of the Breath*

"Most of us have never even considered the gift and value of the breath until something comes in the way of its flow. In *Just Breathe*, Dan succeeds in sharing a lifetime of experience and wisdom in a way that is accessible and practical, but at the same time wakes us up to the magic and mystery of the breath. He makes the simple act of breathing come alive through his passion and deep insight. He guides us to develop a conscious relationship with the breath to optimize every aspect of tour lives. What a gift!"

—Ela Manga, MD, author of *My Energy Codes* and director of Woodlands Spa and Center for Conscious Living, South Africa

"*Just Breathe* is a guide to not only improving your physical, emotional, and psychological health, and your performance, but it is also a guide to raising your consciousness."

—JEAN-LOUIS PORTALES, inventor of the 02Chair

JUST BREATHE

MASTERING BREATHWORK

DAN BRULÉ

FOREWORD BY

TONY ROBBINS

ENLIVEN BOOKS

—

ATRIA

New York   London   Toronto   Sydney   New Delhi

ENLIVEN™

ATRIA

An Imprint of Simon & Schuster, Inc.
1230 Avenue of the Americas
New York, NY 10020

Copyright © 2017 by Daniel Brulé

First Enliven Books/Atria Paperback edition February 2018

For information about special discounts for bulk purchases, please contact Simon &
Schuster Special Sales at 1-866-506-1949 or business@simonandschuster.com.

The Simon & Schuster Speakers Bureau can bring authors to your live event. For
more information or to book an event, contact the Simon & Schuster Speakers
Bureau at 1-866-248-3049 or visit our website at www.simonspeakers.com.

Interior design by Amy Trombat

Manufactured in Italy

20 19 18 17 16 15 14 13 12 11

Library of Congress Cataloging-in-Publication Data is available.

ISBN 978-1-5011-3438-8
ISBN 978-1-5011-6306-7 (pbk)
ISBN 978-1-5011-3439-5 (ebook)

TO PAULINE PEARL, WITH LOVE AND GRATITUDE

CONTENTS

FOREWORD

by Tony Robbins

I've dedicated my life to helping others achieve their peak potential and lead an extraordinary quality of life. And every so often when a teacher comes into my life and teaches me something that expands my own peak experience, I have to share it with others.

That's the case with Dan Brulé, breath master and global teacher of his program Breath Mastery. Dan can help you maximize your performance, reduce stress, boost longevity, optimize health, and ultimately transform your life. He's known as the "Bruce Lee of breathing," because he has drawn the best from every style and school he has explored, and because of his skill, mastery, and dedication to the art and science of breathwork. He's taught tens of thousands of people from around the world—including business leaders, Navy SEALs, athletes, health-care practitioners, and everyday people—looking to improve their health and performance. Dan knows the breathing techniques taught and practiced by ancient yogis and enlightened mystics, elite athletes and warriors, and cutting-edge neuroscientists. Most important, he knows which techniques are best proven to work.

Did you know that 70 percent of the toxins inside our bodies are removed through our lungs? Yet studies show that we're using less and less of our lung capacity. Think about it: When we're stressed out, what do we do? Breathe deep or shallow? It's surprising just how much we hold our breath—think what that does to the body and mind! And what a waste of a natural resource!

Don't waste its power. Be conscious of it. By taking conscious control of your breathing, you harness your thoughts, energy, and body.

People always ask me: "What's the secret to achieving results? The secret to lasting change?" My answer is that you must train yourself to become a master. To become a master at anything takes consistency, commitment, and focus. That's what this book is offering you: the dynamic tools, techniques, and practices to teach, guide, and help you create lasting change in the quality of your life.

It takes 110 percent commitment to reach the level of Breath Mastery that Dan has obtained through decades of study, research, and practice. *Just Breathe* is his definitive handbook, testament, and revelation that once you pay attention to your breath and master its true power, you master your life and your outcomes. This book will show you how. It you want real change that lasts, then you owe it to yourself to start right now with this book in your hands, and master your breath.

—Tony Robbins, 2016

INTRODUCTION: THE BREATH OF LIFE

I've got to keep breathing. It'll be my worst business mistake if I don't.

—STEVE MARTIN

This book introduces to you to the field of *breathwork,* a new and revolutionary approach to self-improvement and self-healing. It shows you how to breathe your way to peak performance, optimum health, and ultimate potential. The exercises, techniques, meditations, and stories here are meant to enlighten and inspire you, and to give you access to the same extraordinary knowledge, skills, and higher states once achieved solely by the great masters, mystics, yogis, saints, gurus, elite athletes, and ancient warriors through years of training.

I've distilled my years of training into this foundational handbook, giving you the optimum tools you need to immediately experience the profound benefits of breathwork. I'll also fill you in on the latest scientific discoveries, the most recent breakthroughs, and the current best practices.

If you are new to breathwork, I can shorten your learning curve, save you lots of time and energy, and help you to create the best foundation for a powerful practice. If you are a seasoned practitioner or a professional breathworker, I can help you deepen and broaden your practice and add to your knowledge and skills so you can take your life and your work to the next level.

The techniques I teach in this book are the same ones I have taught to more than a hundred thousand people—peak performers; life coaches; fitness trainers; psychotherapists; members of the military, active duty and retired; corporate executives; Olympic athletes; elite martial artists; holistic healers; and spiritual teachers and seekers—in more than fifty countries since I started on this path in 1970.

Here are a few testimonials from my clients and students:

Dan coached me through layer after layer of built-up resistance in my body, bringing about an overwhelming yet profoundly peaceful sense of presence of mind, body, and soul.

—————————————

Enormous energy boost! I felt energy in every point in my body.

—————————————

Magnificent! I felt such deep relaxation and bright energy . . . so much aliveness. The "circular breath" and "releasing breath" set me free!

—————————————

It is amazing how much of a difference a few minutes of getting in touch with the breath makes throughout the day. The "sip-sip-sip-POOF" and "sigh" methods you presented for breaking through blockages is extremely helpful.

—————————————

Awesome! I was able to get free from negative thoughts and emotions, and to heal the pain of old traumas.

—————————————

I've had some experiences with Conscious Breathing and am blown away by its transformational effects.

—————————————

Like my clients and students, you will feel how profoundly breathing can change your life and lead to real transformation. The way we breathe in response to pain and pleasure, to stress and change, can make all the difference in the world to our health and well-being, our performance at home and at work, and to our loved ones.

Breathing is the only system in the body that is both automatic and also under our control. That is not an accident of nature, not a coincidence—it's an invitation, an opportunity to take part in our own nature and evolution. There are details in the way you breathe that you probably have never observed or explored, and these details are like doorways that can lead to new and profound abilities. The fact is breathwork is a major skill set if you want to become a high-performing individual and enhance every aspect of your life.

The great masters in every walk of life know the importance of breathing; they use it to prepare and recover and to get through difficult moments and critical situations. Peak performers have a daily breathing practice—their own breathing rituals. It's one of the secrets that give them an edge, put them on top, and keep them in the zone or in a flow state. And this secret source is free! You have the most valuable natural resource right under your nose.

It is time for people in all walks of life to discover, explore, and develop the power and potential of breathwork. Because we all need energy, and we all deal with some form of stress and pressure, pain and fatigue. The conflict and chaos of today's fast-paced living can feel very challenging and even overwhelming. And a victory in the boardroom can be just as important as a victory on the battlefield or on the playing field. Grace, poise, focus, clarity, energy, and calmness are needed in everyday-life situations.

Breathwork promises these benefits and more; it promises to lead you to self-mastery and a transformed life.

What to Expect

Throughout this book, I will be teaching various breathing exercises, techniques, and meditations that I have studied, practiced, and tested, and know will improve and enhance every level of your being. I've organized the chapters under three main categories: body, mind, and spirit. If you need to focus on a particular issue or situation, you can go right to a targeted practice.

Each chapter has real-life stories from breathworkers who are passionate about this work, including parts of my own life. Breathe Now sections guide you through specific breathing techniques, and each chapter ends with a set of simple Everyday Breathing practices. Whether you're waiting in line at the market or stuck in traffic, whether you're feeling scattered, stressed, uninspired, or unmotivated, these quick yet effective "take a breather" moments will do wonders as you roll through your day.

As you practice and experience the breathing techniques in this book, you will quickly realize that a specific breathing exercise, for instance to alleviate physical tension, will inevitably also involve and benefit aspects of your mind and even your spirit. Keep in mind that ultimately breathwork is a life process, connecting and improving every part of you.

Last, I suggest that you start a personal breathing journal or diary. Make notes of what you learn. Write down your favorite techniques and what you are committed to practicing, and keep a record of your experiences and results. This is a great way to see what's working or not; and the journal will be especially helpful for the Twenty-One-Day Breath Mastery Challenge in chapter 6.

1

THE POWER OF BREATH MASTERY

*For breath is life, and if you breathe well you will live
long on earth.*

—SANSKRIT PROVERB

Let me tell you about my awakening to the breath. I was in the
first grade at a Catholic school in New Bedford, Massachusetts.
The pastor of our church made the first of his weekly visits to our
classroom that Friday morning.

We all sat in awe of this very stern-looking old guy dressed in
a long black robe with a bright red cape, holding a leather-bound
Bible, its pages trimmed with gold leaf. We were all afraid. For all we
knew, God could strike us dead if we didn't listen and behave. (Yes, I
am a recovering "Cathaholic.")

Switching back and forth between French and English, he talked
about heaven. That was nice. And he talked about hell—definitely
not nice. He told us how if we were not very, very careful, and if we
did not do exactly as we were told, we would all end up in that terrible place forever! Then he read from the book of Genesis and told us
how: "God took the dust of the earth and formed the body of man;

and breathed into the nostrils of man the breath of life; and man became a living soul."

To say that those words made an impression on me would be a huge understatement. I was smitten! I began to feel uncontrollable and unimaginable excitement at the thought that God was breathing into me. It was the most amazing thing I had ever heard, and I couldn't understand why everyone else wasn't excited about it like me.

I couldn't sit still. I couldn't shut up. I think I was in a state of rapture. I know I became too animated, and I guess I disrupted the class, because I remember the monsignor's hands on my shoulders: he was forcing me to sit back down in my chair.

Either because of him or in spite of him, something in me was definitely awakened that day. I sensed there was something magical, mystical, something wonderful and beautiful about breathing, and no amount of guilt, fear, force, shame, or cajoling was going to change or erase it. This was the spark that lit a fire in me, and to this day, I remain utterly fascinated—more than ever in fact—with breath and breathing, and with the power and potential of breathwork.

From that moment of revelation, my personal path of breathwork took me on an incredible adventure from an X-ray technology program in Boston, and then into the US Navy during the Vietnam War era as an independent hospital corpsman, deep-sea diver, and emergency rescue specialist. I trained CPR and first-aid instructors, EMTs, and other emergency responders; developed the first stress and coping program for the American Red Cross; and designed a master's program called "The Breath as a Tool for Health, Growth, and Change" at Lesley University in Cambridge.

Breathing training led me to study in India with yogi masters; to the Academy of Chinese Medicine in Beijing; and to the Russian Academy of Science in Moscow. I've learned methods of breathing from Zen Buddhism, from Rebirthing with Leonard Orr, from Holotropic Breathwork with Stan Grof, and other sources.

Recently, breathwork led me to Silicon Valley, to the Nissan-Renault Group's Research Labs. This automaker developed a prototype of a car that integrates a breathing feature into the driver's and passenger's seats. A mechanism in the seat, taken from Innovzen's O2 Chair, moves in a way that promotes and supports full, relaxed breathing. It was an honor to present and fun to demonstrate the concept of "onboard breathing" to the CEO and his team. In the next few years as self-driving cars hit the highways, we'll have more free time to focus on other things, like energizing and relaxing ourselves on the way to and from work.

All of these experiences have been the deep well where I've drawn from many different schools and styles of breathing to create a unique and diverse program for breathing training. That's why my martial artist friends call me "the Bruce Lee of breathwork." I'm not saying I'm like Bruce Lee, but one trait we do have in common is the willingness to think outside the box and uncover every stone—to share the best from all of our teachers—and the dedication and dream to teach what we have learned to anyone ready and willing to do the work.

What *Is* Breathwork?

Breathwork is the use of Breath Awareness and Conscious Breathing for healing and growth, personal awakening, and transformation in spirit, mind, and body. All the breathing techniques you'll learn in this book have this definition at their core. Breathwork falls into the field of self-improvement and personal development. It is a self-help, self-healing method in alternative medicine. It is also a key to spiritual purification and self-mastery. It is the most holistic and complementary approach to health care, and it is an essential part of any genuine spiritual development program.

Here is a partial list of settings and situations where breathwork is now being taught and applied, courtesy of Dr. Peter Litchfield (President of the Graduate School of Behavioral Health Services):

Alternative Health Care	Neurofeedback
Anger Management	Nursing
Athletic Coaching	Occupational Therapy
Attention Training	Orthodontics
Biofeedback	Pain Management
Bodywork	Peak Performance Training
Childbirth	Performing Arts
Chiropractic	Personal Coaching
Corporate Training	Physical Therapy
Counseling	Psychology
Dentistry	Public Speaking
Drug Abuse Prevention	Respiratory Therapy
Drug Rehabilitation	Self-regulation Learning
Education (all levels)	Skill Acquisition
Fitness Training	Social Work
Flight Training (aviation)	Speech Therapy
Martial Arts	Stress Management
Medicine	Test Taking
Meditation	Trauma and PTSD
Midwifery	Yoga
Military Training	Zen

More and more people are waking up to the incredible value of breathwork, and they are applying it in their everyday lives at work and at home. Coaches, health-care professionals, counselors, trainers, teachers, and therapists are using it to create breakthroughs for themselves and for those they serve. For spiritual seekers, it's a direct path to spiritual awakening, self-realization, and enlightenment. That's why breathwork is a major skill set that high-performing and successful individuals have mastered—it's the secret ingredient that puts them exactly where they want to be.

I teach breathwork as a formula for personal transformation in which three basic skills or elements are taught:

Awareness (the consciousness factor): The message is "wake up!"
Relaxation (the release factor): The message is "let go!"
Breathing (the energy factor): The message is "take charge!"

I have found that no matter what method is used, or what label is given to it, every miracle event; every healing experience; every positive shift, emotional release, or behavioral change—every bit of growth can be linked to one of these three elements. Real power and magic comes from blending them and simultaneously engaging in these three elements deliberately and consistently. In practice we increase, expand, and refine our awareness. We use the breath to relax more quickly and deeply, and in more situations. And we learn breath control that results in more energy and aliveness, comfort and pleasure, and personal power and resilience.

I also call what I do *breath therapy*, which is based on two key ideas:

1. The breathing system in most people is not functioning at an optimal level. We need to heal it. We need to improve

or restore our breathing capacity, to correct any dysfunctional habits or patterns that inhibit or interfere with the free expression our true nature and full potential.

2. Once our breathing is full and free, healthy and natural, once it is restored or raised to an optimal level, then it automatically becomes a therapeutic tool. The body and breath can be used to heal the mind, and the mind and breath can be used to heal the body. Breathwork can be used to heal attitudes, emotions, and behaviors.

There are five principles of breath therapy. These principles came about as I searched for the answer to this question: "Why do dramatic positive results—even miracles—happen as a result of breathing sessions, and not in other kinds of therapeutic sessions?" The answer to that lies in the application of these five principles:

1. The technique (there are many techniques, each with a certain purpose or effect).
2. The atmosphere in which one practices (physical/psychological/emotional/energetic).
3. The teacher (making use of the "power and purity of our personal presence").
4. The mind of the breather (thoughts, beliefs, attitudes, intentions, desires, will).
5. The "something else" (a mystical or magical factor: luck, grace, timing, readiness).

🌸 BREATHE NOW: HOW ARE YOU BREATHING?

Let's try a quick exercise.

A healthy person should be able to breathe both low in the belly, as well as high in the chest, easily and at will. You should be able to breathe slowly: two or three breaths per minute. And you should be able to breathe quickly: sixty or even 120 breaths per minute. When sitting at rest, your breathing should be low and slow.

How are you breathing? Observe and sense your breathing right now.

Put one hand over your belly and one hand over the center of your chest, and monitor your breathing. How does it feel to breathe? What moves when you breathe? Where does the breath go? Are you a chest breather? A belly breather? Is your breathing fast and shallow, or is it slow and deep? Is it smooth and regular, or choppy and chaotic? Are there pauses in the breathing?

As with any art or skill, the key to excellence or greatness is in understanding and applying the fundamentals. Even the world's greatest musicians practice the scales before a performance. You will go a lot further and a lot faster if you start with the basics and keep returning to them. When it comes to breathwork, there are two basic aspects: Breath Awareness and Conscious Breathing. You can think of these as yin and yang, active and passive aspects of the practice.

Breath Awareness: Being the Breath

Breath Awareness means paying close attention to the breath as you allow it to come and go on its own, by itself. The idea is to simply observe your breathing, watch the breath, witness it. No need to breathe in any particular way. This is the passive aspect. It is the practice of pure awareness applied to breathing.

The awareness we are talking about is meditative awareness. It is not thinking, not judging, not comparing, not analyzing; you are not trying to figure out anything or do anything right. In fact, Breath Awareness is not really something you "do." We are talking about a soft, open state of alertness and presence. **Breath Awareness is a mindfulness practice.** I also call it "breath watching." In fact I use the terms interchangeably. It is attention training. All you need to do is decide to focus on your breathing and to observe it, sense it, moment to moment.

❋ BREATHE NOW: SENSE YOUR BREATHING

Bring your attention to the breath. Focus on your breathing. Sense your breathing. Observe it, listen to it, feel it. Witness it. How do you know you are breathing? What feelings and sensations tell you that you are breathing? Where do those feelings and sensations occur? Where does the breath go when it flows into you? What does it touch? What moves when you breathe? What muscles do you use?

As you become more aware of the breath, you naturally become more aware of other things occurring in your mind and body: thoughts and images, feelings and sensations, perceptions and emotions. You may become more aware of your physical tensions, energetic contractions, habits, patterns, urges, reactions, and inner dialogue.

A very important part of Breath Awareness is simply to witness these various phenomena; notice them without judging, resisting, or attaching to them. If you get distracted by these things, or if your mind wanders off on a tangent, no problem, just return your attention to your breathing and fully focus on the next breath. Look for details in the breathing that perhaps you have never noticed before.

With practice, you will naturally move toward a place of freedom and inner peace, and the realization that nothing is happening *to* you: it is simply happening! You will develop a natural ease and a greater sense of aliveness. Ultimately you will realize that you are always and already free, no matter what you think or how you feel.

Because of the power and potential of this fundamental practice, we are going to spend a lot of time on it, and we'll keep coming back to it, especially in chapter 4, "Breathing to Transform Your Spirit."

Conscious Breathing: Doing the Breathing

The second basic aspect of breathwork is Conscious Breathing. This is where you come in. You are an active participant in the breathing process, more than the witness. Conscious Breathing means that you deliberately control, direct, and regulate the breathing in some way. You give the breathing a certain quality or a specific pattern. You breathe with a conscious intention. You are creative.

With Breath Awareness, the breath breathes you; with Conscious Breathing, you breathe the breath.

An example of a Conscious Breathing exercise is to breathe at a rate of four to eight breaths per minute, which is considered to be a "therapeutic zone" since it has so many naturally therapeutic benefits. So let's begin with an average of six breaths per minute. That means a five-second inhale and a five second exhale.

❋ BREATHE NOW: REGULATE YOUR BREATHING
Breathe in for a count of five seconds, and breathe out for a count of five seconds. Spend some time settling in to this rhythm. Make your

breathing pattern smooth and steady, inhaling for five seconds and exhaling for five seconds. Simple isn't it?

Start by focusing on your breathing. At first simply being aware of it, observe it, then begin to gently bring it under your conscious control. Let the breaths be smooth and steady and rhythmic, inhaling for five seconds and exhaling for five seconds:

Inhale, 2, 3, 4, 5

Exhale, 2, 3, 4, 5

Inhale, 2, 3, 4, 5

Exhale, 2, 3, 4, 5

How do you feel after a few minutes of this practice? If you find it difficult to breathe that slowly, then use a count of two or three or four to start. Or just count faster!

If this rhythm is quite easy, experiment with a count of eight, ten, or twelve, or count more slowly. In any case, don't push, don't force, don't stress, or strain. Relax. Be patient with yourself as you practice.

We will play with many other Conscious Breathing exercises and techniques in the coming chapters, but start with this one to begin a daily practice. Do it first thing in the morning, do it at lunchtime, and do it again before bed. Do it if you find yourself becoming tense or upset, or scattered in your thinking. Remember to:

Inhale, 2, 3, 4, 5

Exhale, 2, 3, 4, 5

Inhale, 2, 3, 4, 5

Exhale, 2, 3, 4, 5

• • •

Practice going back and forth between these two basic elements of breathwork, the fundamental ingredients of breath mastery. **It is essential for us to learn to flow back and forth between active and passive, between doing and being, between breathing the breath and letting the breath breathe us.** In other words, practice both Breath Awareness and Conscious Breathing.

Integrate Breath Awareness and Conscious Breathing into your everyday activities and interactions. For example, when walking or running, pay attention to your breathing or deliberately breathe in rhythm to your footsteps; or when listening to music, notice the quality of your breathing, the effect that the music has on your breathing, or keep the beat with your breath. When stuck in traffic or standing in line at the grocery store, observe your breathing, or gently bring it into this slow, smooth rhythmic pattern of six breaths per minute.

Breathe consciously when you watch a sunset. Use the breath to actually take in the experience. Breathe consciously when someone insults you, praises you, or tells you his or her problems. Begin using your breath to focus or center yourself, to relax or energize yourself. Use it to prepare for important events, to get through challenging tasks, and to recover from stressful experiences.

Get into the habit of observing your breath and taking control of it before, during, and after various activities, events, and interactions. That's the ultimate key to Breath Mastery: turning your daily practice into a way of being. It's especially important to note the changes that occur in your mind and body when you practice breathwork, and track them in your breathing journal.

The way we approach breathwork reflects the way we approach life. By observing your breathing, you can learn a lot about yourself. Sometimes we need to paddle our boat if we expect to get anywhere in life, and sometimes it's better to pull in the oars and let the river of life carry us forward. Sometimes we are called to take charge and sometimes we're called to get out of the way. Sometimes control is necessary and sometimes the call is to surrender. Sometimes we live our life, and at other times life lives us. Sometimes we breathe the breath, and sometimes we let the breath breathe us.

The Three Convergences in Breathwork

Three key elements—what I call "convergences"—create the framework for all breathing methods, styles, and schools. Many breathwork teachers and practitioners have already been applying them intuitively in their own way, because all the benefits of breathwork depend on these three elements for optimum results:

1. Combining consciousness and breathing
2. Combining consciousness and relaxation
3. Combining conscious breathing and complete relaxation

The First Convergence: Combining Consciousness and Breathing

We are breathing all the time, but most of the time we are completely unconscious of it. The breathing is happening, but our consciousness is focused elsewhere. Our awareness is often pushed and pulled and controlled by random unconscious impulses, miscellaneous forces, and other people. The practice of mindful breathing compensates for this, restoring a certain natural power and balance.

When your awareness jumps from one thing to another constantly, your healing energies and creative forces are lost or dissipated. When you bring all your attention to the breathing, your energy begins to accumulate and you develop tremendous personal power. For lack of a better word, "magic" is possible when we bring together consciousness and breathing. For many people, this simple practice is life-changing.

As you begin a daily Conscious Breathing practice, you will dramatically increase your internal awareness as well as your situational awareness. Also, your health, well-being, and performance will be enhanced. When you master Conscious Breathing, you will naturally experience more comfort and pleasure, more success and ease—in body and mind, in your intimate relationships, and in your professional life.

The Second Convergence: Combining Consciousness and Relaxation

Consider this: when you are in your most relaxed state, you are literally sleeping. You actually sleep through the most relaxing moments of your life! You are unconscious in those moments when you are most relaxed, so you have probably never had a waking experience of pure, deep, and total relaxation.

You have to get out of the way for your body to relax and rejuvenate itself. Your ordinary consciousness—filled and busy as it is with all its incessant mental activity—interferes in the body's ability to relax. Thus nature sees to it that you disappear for a while every night. Having you go unconscious seems to be the only way your body can take a break from your head tripping! Slumping on a couch, drinking beer, and watching TV is a very poor substitute for genuine relaxation.

Being wide awake and totally relaxed at the same time is so rare that when it occurs during a breathing session, most people describe it as a peak religious experience, a peace that passes understanding. They describe the experience as bliss or ecstasy, a feeling of pure, causeless joy. They inevitably resort to spiritual or religious terms to describe what is actually a very basic, yet profound human experience.

When you master this second convergence in breathwork—bringing together full consciousness and complete relaxation—you touch a place in yourself, you open to a state that all the great masters and saints lived in and lived from. You get a taste of the life lived by the Buddha, Jesus, Lao-tzu, Krishna, and all the other sublime teachers.

The Third Convergence: Combining Conscious Breathing and Complete Relaxation

This is a high art and a transformational skill: the merging of peace and power. Master it, and you will discover, experience, and accomplish things that the average person can only dream of.

Usually when people breathe in a powerful way, they don't relax. And when they relax completely, they don't breathe. The more they breathe, the less they relax; the more they relax, the less they breathe. This is the common dilemma and the normal experience of people who have not mastered the art of breathwork. The idea is to turn it all around so the more you breathe, the more you relax, and the more you relax, the more you breathe. Stop sacrificing one for the other and you will enter the ranks of the great saints and yogis, the famous artists and legendary warriors.

Here we apply the principle of economy: we focus on breathing fully and freely, deeply and powerfully, all while using as little muscular effort or activity as possible. We engage in deliberate relaxation even as we practice breathing deeper, faster, and more powerful breaths.

Combining full, free breathing and complete relaxation with great awareness is the secret that leads to the most empowering and enlightening benefits in breathwork. It is the door to what we call peak, flow, or transcendent states. It can be described as an "energized calm" or a "dynamic peace." You owe it to yourself to master this third and key convergence in breathwork.

The Three Convergence Reminders

---

1. Practicing the first convergence means practicing mindful breathing or Breath Awareness. You're learning to let the breath breathe you.

2. The second convergence is about becoming conscious of the tensions in your body and eliminating unnecessary muscular activity. It's especially important to relax the accessory breathing muscles.

3. The third convergence is about combining powerful breathing and deep relaxation in a conscious and creative way.

2

BREATHING TO TRANSFORM YOUR BODY

Breath is the bridge which connects life to consciousness,
which unites your body to your thoughts.

—THICH NHAT HANH

In June 1970 I was in boot camp, where they made you run everywhere all the time. I quickly learned how to pace my breathing in rhythm to my footsteps to be able to keep up and even stay ahead. You also shut up and stand still a lot (often while they shout insults at you). It's normal to hold your breath in those moments, and had I known then what I know now, I would have breathed quietly and consciously instead. That would have allowed me to take in their instruction without getting frazzled or feeling intimidated

We shouted all the time. "Yes, sir!" "No, sir!" "I can't hear you!" "Yes, Sir!" "I still can't hear you!" *"Yes, sir!"* I shouted so loud one time that I tore my vocal cords and lost my voice. It was the strangest thing: I could only shout or whisper. I had nothing in between—which worked out perfectly for the military, because they wanted you to either yell or be silent. So no one even noticed my problem, and the last thing I wanted to do was ask to go to the hospital. Suck it up. "Grin and bear it" was the unspoken rule.

I was assigned to the Naval Hospital Corps School out of boot camp, and on the first day I was put into a special accelerated program. Four of us were selected because of our previous college or medical training, I suppose. Together we finished thirty-six weeks of Hospital Corps School in less than three weeks. Then we spent another three weeks qualifying for all the practical skills: physical exams, bandaging, splinting, drawing blood, giving injections, and sticking things down each other's throats, into each other's noses and ears, and up each other's butts—basically getting skilled and comfortable with just about everything we might be called upon to do out in the field or in a hospital.

At the end of the training, I was offered a special advancement incentive: it was called "Push Button E-4." In exchange for extending my enlistment from four to six years, I could immediately advance to petty officer third class, a rate and a pay grade that normally took a good sailor at least two years to earn. I had been in the navy for only four months.

I was now officially an independent duty hospital corpsman. My first assignment was at a dispensary across the river from the Naval Academy in Annapolis, Maryland. I was put in charge of my own X-ray department. On the first day, I took an inventory and did a detailed inspection. I found a very serious problem: the facility did not meet the most basic radiation safety standards. There was no lead shielding anywhere in the building.

Since there was no X-ray work to do, and we had nine corpsmen working (on the busiest day, four of us could easily handle the workload), I was getting bored and began to spend time with the crew of the USS *Alvin,* the navy's first deep-sea submersible. I began to work with local civilian authorities to train first responders, and I led safety and rescue programs and health inspections. I took every ambulance call that came in, and over the next eighteen months, I taught first aid and CPR to just about every fireman and policeman in the states of Maryland and Delaware.

When my two-year assignment at the naval station was up, I had advanced to petty officer second class. I was now an E-5 (an enlisted rank), and I had orders for the aircraft carrier USS *John F. Kennedy*. I was being transferred to what was basically a floating city with as many as five thousand crewmembers. It was the last place I wanted to be, and the last thing I wanted to do. I had grown way too comfortable with my independence, and joining the "regular navy" felt like a prison sentence.

I called Washington and requested that I be sent anywhere else, assigned to anything else. "Anything?" the person on the phone asked me.

"Yes, sir. Anything," I said. Thus I was assigned to Special Operations: Deep Sea Diving School. It came with a juicy raise (they called it "hazardous duty pay").

The combination of medical skills, deep-sea diving, and salvage and rescue training would make me a member of a very unique and elite group in one of the oldest and proudest traditions in the navy—a medical deep-sea diving technician. I would learn underwater welding and ship salvage, receive demolition training, and be given the opportunity to do a whole lot of things very few people ever got the chance to do.

The guy on the phone gave me the impression that I really didn't know what I was getting myself into. He said, "Hey, want some advice?"

I said, "Sure!"

"You've got two months before you report in for the program. You better start running everywhere, all the time, and with ninety pounds of gear on your back, or you won't make it through the first two weeks."

I thought: *Hmmm . . . physical training.* "I'm up for that!"

I was the champion pool player on the base at the time, and befriended the base boxing champion. He approached me with a proposition: I teach him to play pool and he teaches me to box.

I thought it would be a great way to supplement my physical training and so I agreed. I really liked the first couple of sessions with him, learning some basic stances and moves and hitting the bag. I had no idea there was so much to learn. It was kind of fun, and it was a real workout. I also loved his coaching around the breath. Every punch had a breath sound!

Then we had our first sparring session. And every time he hit me, or even pretended to hit me, I would close my eyes. I wanted to run away or curl up in a ball like a baby. Every time he hit me somewhere, I would instinctively move to protect that place, so he would hit me in another unprotected place; or he would just knock my arms out of the way and hit me in the same place again! He kept pointing it out and calling me hopeless.

"You're afraid to get hit! Man, you have to learn to love it."

"Love it? What are you talking about? Nobody loves getting hit."

"I do. I love it!" (And he really did. He was crazy that way.)

This went on every day, and for a while it didn't seem like a very good trade. We would meet at lunch and he would beat me up for an hour; then after work I would play pool with him. But then at one point I realized that I was not afraid so much of pain as I was of intensity, and I began to notice that many of his punches really didn't hurt. They were intense, sort of stunning, more numbing than painful. I began to control my breathing to keep from getting the wind knocked out of me. I also began to pay more attention to his breathing, and started to see how it helped me to sense things about him.

My fear started losing its grip on me. I was able to keep my eyes open, even as his big, fat glove came straight into my face. I began to sense when and what was coming. By paying attention, I knew what he was going to do from how he planted his feet, or from the angle he tried to get on me. I began to get a sense of his rhythms: one, two; one, two . . . one, two, three; one, two . . . one, two; one, two three . . .

Then one day as I walked across the street to the gym, preparing to get beat up again, I stopped to take a few breaths to prepare and commit. I was suddenly struck with such a clear and conscious sense of a new and expanded level of being present and awake.

I took in a very conscious breath, and I felt it go to every cell of my body. That breath was delicious, and it gave me goose bumps. I took another one and it felt even better than the first. I was elated! I took another breath and felt the emotions turn into streaming physical energy that made me wiggle my toes with pleasure.

I was moved to look up and I stretched my arms to the sky. And as I breathed in, it felt as if I was taking in the power of God. I could feel the earth under my feet, loving me. Even the trees and the clouds and the birds seemed to love me. The grace of God was surrounding me. With every breath, I felt more and more energy and aliveness coursing through me. And so I kept on breathing, taking in one breath after the next without stopping.

My eyes saw everything in Technicolor; it was as if my consciousness was opening and expanding with every breath I took. When I looked around, I could see the energy in the air—tiny particles of light were moving, dancing, and swirling everywhere. I thought, *So this is what cats are seeing when they seem to stare into empty space!*

A very special feeling took over me as I crossed the street that day toward the boxing ring, and it has never really left me. I often return to that moment in order to remember or reawaken to who I am or how I can be. And to do that, all I have to do is relax, focus on my breathing, and feel.

As we started sparring, I began to look forward to getting hit! It's hard to explain, but I was actually beginning to enjoy it—the energy and intensity of it. The pain—if that is the only word we have for it—just made me feel more alive. He started taking more shots than usual at my stomach and lower rib cage, in rapid machine-gun fashion, and I found that I could meet his blows with my energy, or I could absorb them with my breath.

He began to turn up the heat. I realized he had been holding back on me out of kindness or something all this time, and now I began to feel just how hard this guy could hit. And I could sense that he was enjoying really letting go into his full-on violent urges.

For a short moment his power was frightening. It rocked me; I was in over my head, and I sensed the urge to curl up or run away. But instead, I tucked my chin down, bit my mouthpiece, planted my back foot, and leaned into his attack. I found that by focusing on the center of his chest in an open, soft way, I could see all of him, from head to toe.

When I saw a punch coming, I actually threw myself at it. And I started to plan my own attack, looking for targets and openings. I decided to lure him in. I deliberately gave him an angle that he liked, knowing he would use the opportunity to fire off his favorite weapon: a right hook to my head.

I felt exactly when he was about to unload, and as he did, I didn't even try to block it. I came up from underneath with a powerful left of my own, right into the side of his ribs. As they say: I beat him to the punch.

I put the power of my breath behind that shot, and I heard what sounded like a stick in the mud breaking, and he went down like a sack of potatoes. I was shocked. It took him a few minutes just to get onto one knee. I was already taking my gloves off; I knew he was hurt bad. When I helped him to his feet, he couldn't straighten up, and he was having trouble breathing.

At the hospital, we learned that I had broken two of his ribs, and one of them punctured his lung! I felt so bad sitting by his bed that night. And even though it hurt, he insisted on hugging me, and as he did, he said: "Man, you are one dangerous son of a bitch!" I felt like the president had given me the Medal of Honor that day, and I felt like I was ready for anything. It provided me the kind of confidence I needed for what came next.

• • •

In the navy diving world of the seventies, there seemed to be an acceptance of crude, vulgar language, and of blatantly racist and sexist attitudes. Running around the base every morning we would sing: "Eat, bite, fuck, chew! I'm a deep-sea diver, who the hell are you?" Deep-sea divers were supposed to be the toughest guys on the block, and to a few of them, that meant going out of their way to look for fights. There I was, a pacifist at heart, playing the animal thug game with them, both loving and hating it.

Before you are accepted into diving school, you have to pass a physical exam and report for an orientation dive. That's when a lot of guys discover that they have claustrophobia. They put you in the full deep-sea rig—lead shoes, lead weights, brass helmet, and breastplate— and throw you over the side of the barge. When it was my turn, I found myself upside down stuck in the mud at the bottom of the Anacostia River, with water leaking into my suit and helmet.

At first, all I could focus on was catching my breath. As soon as I got it under control, I felt good. Then my next goal was maneuvering around to get upright. I laughed at my predicament and how silly I must have looked from a distance. It turned out to be fun until I became short of breath again, and realized I had to figure out how to regulate my air control and exhaust valve.

Once I got the hang of it, my attention turned to the darkness. It was pitch dark, and for some strange reason, I liked it. The world on the surface, my past—everything just disappeared. I felt at home. By the time I climbed back up the ladder onto the deck of that barge, I was as thrilled as I was exhausted.

The physical and psychological training in medical deep-sea diving school was intense, and the work was extremely challenging: physics, respiratory chemistry, diving medicine, mixing gases, salvage and rescue, firefighting, demolition training, along with lots of time under water in the dark, alone or with a buddy. Every day brought a new adventure. One consistently predictable thing was morning physical training. It was always a struggle for me. I never really enjoyed those workouts. They were boring and tedious, not to mention tiring, but I forced myself to tolerate them.

One morning run, we did a lot more jumping jacks, push-ups, chin-ups, and sit-ups than usual. After a little too much partying the night before, I was having a particularly tough time of it, and I was almost relieved when we started our run. But the relief didn't last long. Three miles into our five-mile run, it felt like torture. I began to wonder if I would even make it. I hung in there, and was so relieved when we finally approached the finish point.

But my relief turned to despair when Youngblood, our trainer, didn't even slow down at the five-mile marker. In fact, he picked up the pace! I hesitated, and felt myself slowing down, and if one of the guys hadn't pushed me from behind in that moment, I would have given up. This was a test, we found out later, and sure enough, several guys failed. They dropped out or were cut from the class that day. And I came very close to being one of them.

What saved me that day was Kane, one of my diving buddies who saw me slowing down and began to run beside me, encouraging me. That moral support and his presence helped for a few minutes, but then it wasn't enough. My body wanted to quit; it felt like lead. And my mind was not helping. It wanted me to listen to my body and quit. But out of the height of my despair, I heard Kane shouting at me: "You can do it. Let's breathe together." And we did, with him setting the pace: breathing in for three steps and breathing out for three steps, in for three steps and out for three steps. That total, single-minded focus on my breathing was like magic. It took my attention off everything else: my pain, fatigue, and negative mental dialogue.

Energy seemed to come out of nowhere, and I was only a few steps behind the leader when we finished the run. Afterward, they made us do more push-ups, chin-ups, and sit-ups. By then I was determined to do whatever was called for. I continued the breathing, moving my breath with conscious force in sync to the repetitive exercises.

A few months later, I was officially a medical deep-sea diving technician, and I was in the best shape of my life. Thirty-seven of us started the program, and six of us completed it. I wore my diving pin with pride.

• • •

You don't need to be a deep-sea diver or a professional boxer to apply Breath Awareness and Conscious Breathing to your life. The lessons I learned during those years have helped me in many other situations, and they can help you meet your unique life challenges. For example, if you need to focus on something, start by focusing on your breath. **If you need to control yourself—your mind, body, emotions, posture, or behavior—then start by getting control of your breathing.**

I learned that when we breathe together, when we synchronize our breathing, we connect in a certain subtle way. When we breathe together, we tend to think alike, to react at the same time and in the same way to the same things. If you breathe together with those you love or those with whom you work, you will begin to read each other's minds and give each other energy. Bonds are strengthened. Intimacy is enhanced. Teamwork goes to a higher level.

The lesson here is that whenever you think you are reaching a limit, you need to become aware of your breathing and breathe consciously. It's almost like a mind trick: when you are focused on your breathing, when you are breathing consciously, then you're not focused on what would normally limit or control your thinking. When you focus on your breath instead, something new, something else, is possible.

Breathing Together: Team Building

We can take our individual practice to new levels by breathing together. When we breathe together, sharing a heartfelt intent or a common vision, we can create a deeper connection and generate an intuitive force that is extremely powerful.

Throughout history, when small, close-knit groups of people prepared to set out to change the world together, or their small piece of it, they would form a circle, hold hands, or lock arms. They might pray, chant, dance, or breathe together in ritual fashion. The simple act of repeating a vow, reciting a prayer, or just shouting together would result in their synchronizing their breath in that moment.

Could it be that the closeness that groups feel has something to do with sharing the same breath? Could it be part of the reason people feel good after group meditation, praying, singing or chanting a hymn or mantra out loud together? Or feeling more energy and confidence from moving together, from dancing or running as one united force?

Teams of all kinds—from sports, artistic performance, business and finance, military and security, schools, and ordinary families—can use the power of breath to unite and be more in tune with each other under a common cause or shared purpose. People who work together, begin a mission together, or who simply want to celebrate their connection, can use the breath in this way: using a simple two-two pattern, inhaling for a count of two and exhaling for a count of two.

Breathing together may have benefits that truly bring success in life, business, and beyond for you and those with whom you live, work, and play.

How Breathwork Affects Your Body

How do we understand the connection between controlling our breath and the powerful effects that it produces? A good place to start is with the autonomic nervous system, which regulates all the automatic functions of the body. It is also the main regulator in our stress-response system. The autonomic nervous system is made up of two counterbalancing parts: the sympathetic nervous system (SNS) and the parasympathetic nervous system (PNS). The sympathetic system goes into action when we are under stress or enduring a challenge, or have to mobilize to get something we want or to avoid something harmful.

When the challenge or danger has passed, what is supposed to happen is that the sympathetic system quiets down, while its counterpart, the parasympathetic system, comes online and begins to counteract all the effects of the "fight-or-flight" response. For example, the sympathetic system speeds up our heart rate and respiration, and the parasympathetic slows them both down and triggers our natural "rest and digest, restore and repair" functions. The parasympathetic system restores energy reserves and reduces inflammation.

But what happens all too often is that our sympathetic system stays highly active instead of returning to baseline, while our parasympathetic system is underactive, especially in people who suffer chronic stress or trauma. That's when we see people experience inappropriate overreactions and difficulty relaxing or calming down; they feel unsafe and stuck in a defensive mode. So, how can breathing help correct this imbalance?

Dr. Richard P. Brown, associate clinical professor of psychiatry at Columbia University, has been using a wide variety of breathing practices for the past fifty years, first in martial arts, Zen meditation, and aikido (fourth dan), then as a teacher of yoga, qigong, and meditation. Dr. Patricia Gerbarg, a graduate of Harvard Medical School and the Boston Psychoanalytic Society and Institute and assistant clinical professor of psychiatry at New York Medical College, became interested in the neuropsychology of breathing practices over fifteen years ago. She and Dr. Brown have been exploring how specific breathing practices can reduce the activity of the SNS and boost the activity of the PNS. For information on their work and publications, visit www .breath-body-mind.com.[1]

One key to the puzzle comes from the work of the neuroanatomist

Dr. Stephen Porges, distinguished university scientist at the Kinsey Institute, Indiana University Bloomington. Dr. Porges formulated the Polyvagal Theory based on his discovery of three evolutionary stages in our autonomic system that help us deal with the demands of life.[2]

Most of the pathways of the PNS travel through two large nerves: the vagus nerves that exit from the brain stem, one on each side, and continue down throughout the body, sending branches to all internal organs. About 20 percent of these pathways send messages from the brain down to the body (efferent) to regulate the organs. About 80 percent of the pathways bring information from the body up to the brain (afferent)—millions of bits of information every millisecond, telling the brain what is going on inside the body. Our perception of this sensory information from inside the body is called interoception.

Dr. Brown and Dr. Gerbarg applied Dr. Porges's discoveries to understanding how breath practices work. They explain that the respiratory system has millions of receptors: chemical receptors, pressure receptors, and stretch receptors. With every breath in and out, microscopic stretch receptors fire in the walls of millions of alveoli (the air-filled sacs inside the lungs). Studies have shown that when we change our pattern of breathing, we change the interoceptive messages going from the respiratory system to the brain.

Where is all this information going, and what does it do inside the brain? Dr. Brown and Dr. Gerbarg have gathered a good deal of evidence through electronic vagal nerve stimulation, brain-imaging studies, and clinical trials to support their theory that this information reaches the brain centers that process and regulate our emotions, perceptions, judgments, thoughts, and behaviors. They agree with Dr. Porges and Dr. Sue Carter, director of the Kinsey Institute and Rudy Professor of Biology at Indiana University Bloomington, whose recent work indicates that the activity of the vagal PNS system has significant effects on our abilities to trust, love, connect, bond, be intimate, communicate emotionally, and feel empathy. According to Dr. Gerberg, "Because breathing has such a strong impact on our thoughts and feelings, it provides a portal through which we can send messages through our own nervous systems to quiet our minds, reduce defensive overreactivity, and enable us to feel safe, close, loving, and loved."[3]

Based on their studies of people with severe anxiety, depression, and post-traumatic stress disorder (PTSD), including survivors of mass disasters, Dr. Brown and Dr. Gerberg teach a form of Conscious Breathing called "coherent breathing": breathing gently and naturally through the nose at a rate of four and a half to six breaths per minute, using a chime tone to pace the breathing. To this they add other techniques to strengthen and balance the SNS and PNS.[4]

As a team, Dr. Brown, Dr. Gerberg, and their colleagues formulate and test theories about how breathing may be used to relieve stress, anxiety, depression, and PTSD as well as stress-related medical problems, such as inflammatory bowel disease. In one of their books, *The Healing Power of the Breath*, a CD helps teach the breathing practices to readers.[5]

When we speed up or slow down our breathing, we activate the sympathetic and parasympathetic responses. (Any kind of breathing, not just "diaphragmatic breathing" affects the vagal nerves.) By controlling our breath, we can willfully influence the brain and the autonomic nervous system and literally change our mind-body state. **By changing the pattern of our breathing, we change the pattern of the information being sent to the brain.** In other words, how often, how fast, and how much you inflate your lungs directly affects the brain and how it operates.

Breathing affects every organ, system, and function in the body.

Every physiological, psychological, and emotional state has a corresponding breathing pattern. When you change one, the other changes. Therefore, Conscious Breathing techniques have the potential to transform the quality of your life on every level and on a day-to-day basis.

When we are focused on a challenging task, when we have too much on our minds, when we are worried about the kids, school, money, or aging parents, we are functioning in the sympathetic zone. Our bodies are producing more free radicals, and we are not able to relax or to feel close and cuddly. We also tend to make snap judgments and be more reactive, and we are less flexible, relaxed, and creative.

Conscious Breathing can balance and counteract all that. Breathwork can become a powerful and natural alternative or adjunct in dealing with post-traumatic stress, anxiety disorders, and many other conditions.

Your Heart Rate and Longevity

Conscious Breathing can increase heart rate variability, which improves a range of symptoms such as stress, anxiety, cardiovascular disease, fatigue, obesity, depression, and aging.

Dr. David O'Hare has been practicing general medicine for over thirty years. He graduated from the Faculty of Medicine of Marseilles, France, and he also holds a postgraduate degree in cognitive and behavioral therapy. He has been practicing and researching the link between heart-rate variability and breathing since 1977.

Heart rate variability, or HRV, refers to the natural tendency of the heart to speed up and slow down with each breath. Having higher HRV is a sign of a healthy heart and an indicator of overall well-being. Many researchers like Dr. O'Hare have been studying and bringing awareness of this phenomenon to the world.

Yogis, Taoist monks, and others are known to be able to control various so-called involuntary physiological processes in the body: heart rate, brain states, and so on. Dr. O'Hare teaches a very simple and specific breathing practice that allows anyone to take more control over their health and to begin to develop some of those same abilities. The title of his book, *Heart Coherence 365,* describes both the practice formula and the benefits.

Dr. O'Hare explains: "When we breathe in, the heart speeds up. The mechanism is complex; it has to do with inhibiting the parasympathetic nervous system (the brake). It is like lifting our foot off the brake on a downhill slope; the car accelerates. When we exhale, the heart slows, like reapplying the brakes on a downhill slope; the car slows down."[6]

Breathing gives us a way to hack into our own brain and nervous system!

High HRV is linked to longevity, and it is inversely proportionate to stress. The more stressed you are, the less your heart speeds up and slows down with every breath. The less stressed you are, the greater the range of your HRV. When you are in the zone, it is at peak or optimal variability.

Various things reduce HRV: aging; chronic illnesses like diabetes, cardiovascular disease, cancer, obesity, stress, anxiety, depression, tobacco consumption, or insomnia; and lack of exercise.

We normally measure heart rate in beats per minute, and we assume that a regular, steady rhythm is good. In fact, a steady, regular heart rate is the last thing you want! When we measure the heart rate in milliseconds, we find that the time between two heartbeats is never the same.

Imagine a tennis player waiting for her opponent's serve. She doesn't take a solid stance, and she doesn't move in a predictable direction or in a repetitive or mechanical way. She keeps moving, jumping, randomly shifting from one foot to the other. This is how she remains ready and able to respond in any direction at any time to whatever comes her way.

A healthy heart is always adjusting to the internal and external environment. A healthy heart rate is irregular! It is resilient, responsive, adapting moment to moment. It is alive. So don't worry and don't be nervous if you notice your heart speeding up or slowing down. It is doing its job of serving you.

Slow-paced breathing increases HRV, supports the heart, and improves stress resilience. The lesson here is to practice breathing at a rate of six breaths per minute. When you do, an interesting phenomenon called "heart resonance" is produced in as little as five minutes.

Heart coherence refers to the continuous fluctuations in the heart rate. It is associated with a positive state or mood—a feeling of inner balance and centeredness—alert yet relaxed, energized yet calm. There are a number of ways to create heart coherence. There are cognitive methods such as visualization, for example; and practices like tai chi, yoga, regular exercise, meditation, also increase it. When we imagine or remember a pleasant event or a wonderful experience, the heart tends toward coherence.

You can create heart coherence using emotional methods, such as when you generate feelings like love and affection, compassion, goodwill, and gratitude. And you can use evocation methods such as repeating affirmations, declarations, positive verbal statements, prayers, mantras, and so on.

However, by far the quickest and most effective way to guarantee heart coherence is through Conscious Breathing. Heart coherence is at its maximum when a resonant frequency of four and a half to six respiratory cycles per minute is attained. In other words, when you breathe at a rate of four and a half to six breaths per minute, you trigger heart coherence.

Studies show measurable benefits with just five minutes of paced breathing at a rate of six breaths per minute, three times per day. You can reduce heart rate, blood pressure, and cortisol levels (that's the stress hormone) by up to 20 percent!

Six breaths per minute means five-second inhales and five-second exhales. When you breathe in this way, you get a handle on your autonomic nervous system and influence your physiology in a very positive way. The benefits include a reduction in cortisol levels and increases in oxytocin, dopamine, serotonin as well as an increase in brain alpha waves. All of these benefits can be produced in just five minutes, and they can last for up to four hours or more. Not bad for five minutes of a simple breathwork technique!

There is a catch: your breathing practice is only effective when it becomes a daily ritual, like showering or brushing your teeth. That's what produces the permanent, ongoing benefits, and it's how we produce higher levels of fitness and performance, not to mention a healthier heart and a longer life.

After seven to ten days of practice, the measurable benefits are significant, and they last for several weeks after you stop. But why stop? The benefits only accumulate when you choose to make this practice a regular part of your day. So why not start today?

❋ BREATHE NOW: HEART RATE VARIABILITY PRACTICE

Three times per day

Six breaths per minute

Five minutes duration

Make your in-breaths and your out-breaths last for five seconds each. There is an imperceptible pause between inhales and exhales. In this way, you create heart coherence and heart resonance. (See Heart Rate Variability Reminders on page 37 for clarification of these terms.)

Sit straight and strong, but relaxed and at ease. It's easier to breathe fully and freely and to create heart coherence if you are sitting or standing upright.

Create a conscious intention before each session. State it as an affirmation, an assertion, a command, or a prayer. For example: "I am strengthening my ability to survive and thrive till I'm a hundred and five!" Or "Every conscious breath makes me stronger, healthier, and more alive!"

Breathe in for five seconds: through your nose, focusing on sending the breath low into your belly. (It's okay to breathe in through your mouth if that feels more comfortable, interesting, or enjoyable.)

Breathe out for five seconds: through your nose, or perhaps through pursed lips as if you are blowing through a straw to make bubbles in your drink, or by making a *shhhh* sound. Some people like to hum on the exhale. That also works beautifully. Do what feels comfortable or enjoyable.

Be fully mindful of each breath when you practice. Focus 100 percent on the subtle sensations of breathing. It is not a thinking process, it is a feeling process. This is how we access our unconscious autonomic system and take control of so-called involuntary functions.

Do your first five-minute practice session as soon as you wake up in the morning, before doing anything else (except perhaps using the toilet). Do this first session before drinking coffee or having breakfast. It is the most important session of the day. Make it a priority.

Do your second five-minute session about four hours later, just before lunch. This midday session clears away stress and rebalances the nervous system after a hectic morning. It also prepares your system for digestion, and it helps prevent afternoon drowsiness.

Do your third session at the end of your workday, perhaps in your car when you arrive home or before starting your evening. Practice breathing six breaths per minute for five minutes to help you shift from work mode to family life. On especially long or busy days, you can add one more session, about an hour before sleeping—for example about 10 P.M. if you go to bed at eleven.

Remember the formula for breathing at resonant frequency:

> Three times per day
> Six breaths per minute
> Five minutes duration

To reinforce the breathing signal, focus on your heart. You can even put your hand(s) over your heart. Focus on positive emotions, wonderful images, and powerful intentions.

Use the *shhhh* sound on the exhale, or purse your lips as if blowing through a straw to make bubbles in your drink.

Do one or two minutes of practice before an important meeting or activity, to calm and focus yourself, and to prepare physiologically. Do it when you become emotionally upset or offended.

Breathing at resonant frequency helps not only you, it influences the hearts of those who are close to you. Practice it when your children become agitated. Try it when your baby cries, or when your spouse is angry, upset, or in pain.

Heart Rate Variability Reminders

1. Heart rate variability (HRV) is the ability of the heart to accelerate and decelerate in relation to changes in your internal

and external environment. The range of this variability reflects your capacity to adapt to and cope with change.

2. Heart chaos is the natural state of the HRV curve. The heart accelerates and decelerates as it adapts moment to moment to our internal and external environments.

3. Heart coherence is a specific state of increased heart rate variability induced by paced breathing. It represents inner harmony and balance, and it results in many beneficial effects on health and well-being.

4. Heart resonance is a specific state of heart coherence attained when breathing consciously and deeply at a frequency of six times per minute.

For more information about Dr. O'Hare's breathing program, visit: http://justbreathe365.com/.

The Iceman: Energy and Immune Boost

The Iceman's breathing technique will give a powerful boost to your energy levels and strengthen your immune system. It will improve concentration, circulation, mood, and take your performance to a higher level.

He has climbed Mount Everest and Mount Kilimanjaro in his underwear; he's run full marathons through high deserts without food or water. He holds twenty Guinness World Records, and his name is Wim Hof.

He is known as "the Iceman" because he loves extreme cold: he's voluntarily been buried up to his neck in ice for almost two hours, which brings his skin temperature down to almost freezing, yet his core temperature remains normal—in fact, he can raise it by one degree. In addition to his ability to withstand extreme temperatures, under laboratory conditions, he has been injected with endotoxins, flu-type bacteria, with no ill effects whatsoever. In other words, he can influence his immune system and autonomic nervous system, and he teaches others to do the same.

How does he do it? With breathwork, of course! Wim meditates and practices yoga, and his method also involves training in gradual cold exposure. By bringing this all together, he has learned to overcome extreme conditions and to supercharge his immune system.

His basic method involves alternating between deep breathing and breath holding, a simple yet very powerful practice. With focus and commitment, you too can learn to control your immune system and autonomic nervous system to improve your circulation, boost your energy levels, improve concentration and focus, sleep better, put yourself in a more positive mood, and take your performance to a higher level.

Here is one of Wim's basic breathing techniques:

1. Take a few long, slow, deep, gentle breaths to focus, relax, and prepare.

2. Take in thirty or forty deep, full breaths and let the exhales out without any force. (Breathe in through your nose and out through your mouth, or breathe in and out through your mouth.)

3. Take in one more long, deep breath, let the exhale go, and hold your breath out (don't breathe in). When you feel a strong urge to breathe or your diaphragm begins to flutter, take in a full inhale and hold it in for ten or fifteen seconds, then let go, exhale, and relax. That's it! Do three rounds of this exercise, two or three times every day. Don't force it. And you will see that over a few weeks your breathing ease and capacity will increase dramatically, you will be able to comfortably hold your breath for longer periods, and you will begin to notice many health and performance benefits—guaranteed.

As an advanced practice, or as an athletic experiment, you can do push-ups or squats or some other repetitive exercise while holding your breath on the third round. Most people are surprised to learn that they can do more reps than usual during that final breath-holding phase.

Another important piece of Wim's method involves the use of gradual cold exposure, and he has taken his love of the cold to amazing extremes. He advises beginners to start by simply taking a cold shower every morning. Or, if you need to start more slowly, take a warm shower and end it with a cold rinse of about a minute.

To learn more about Wim and his work, visit www.wimhof method.com/justbreathe.

Some Facts About Hyperventilation

Hyperventilation, also called "overbreathing," can be learned or occur reflexively, and ironically, it can leave you feeling breathless.

When hyperventilation occurs reflexively or happens unintentionally and becomes out of control, it can trigger anxiety or panic, The reverse can also happen—anxiety or panic triggers the hyperventilation. When you hyperventilate, you blow off too much carbon dioxide (CO_2). In body fluids, such as the blood, carbon dioxide forms carbonic acid, which regulates acid-base balance, literally from breath to breath. Therefore, dysfunctional breathing can very quickly disturb your acid-base balance, resulting in respiratory alkalosis, an undesirable rise in blood plasma pH. This can result in symptoms such as tingling or numbness of the lips, muscle spasms in the hands and feet, belching, and chest pain. Hyperventilation can also radically reduce blood flow to the brain, resulting in symptoms such as headaches, confusion, weakness, dizziness, agitation, palpitations, fainting, and even seizures.

Paradoxically, when hyperventilation is learned and intentional in your breathing practice, it can be an effective way to overcome deep fears and transform emotions, especially feelings of limitations, blocks, and old traumas. It is a method of spiritual purification and a powerful healing and creative practice when used properly. Using hyperventilation consciously in breathing training develops your ability to relax through uncomfortable feelings and to overcome physiological, emotional, and psychological barriers.

The Super Human: Breath Holding and PTSD

The breathwork techniques here will boost your energy levels and improve relaxation, concentration, and sleep. If you suffer from chronic stress, depression, or especially PTSD, this is a great complementary practice to integrate into your healthcare program.

Stig Severinsen is a modern-day yogi. He is a Danish free diver who holds a number of world records, including the longest free dive under ice (250 feet), and the longest breath hold underwater: twenty-two minutes. He is an extreme athlete and also has a PhD in biology and medicine. Many people know of him through the Discovery Channel documentary about him called *Stig Severinsen: The Man Who Doesn't Breathe.* They also chose him as the "Ultimate Super Human" on *Superhuman Showdown.* Stig believes that the breath provides a link between the body and mind by which we can control the stress response. He loves to challenge scientific dogmas, and his passion is testing the limits of human potential.

He sees breathwork as an art form. And just as in any art, he says, we need to put in the time and practice to get extraordinary results. For him, the first step is consciousness: "Just stop and meditate on your breath. Focus on your breathing. Listen to the breathing."

Stig sees breathwork as a spiritual discipline. He says that breathwork is a way of training our intuitive side and tuning into our hearts: it awakens our ability to pick up on other people's energy, and it even leads to the awakening and development of psychic abilities. He says it allows us to expand the mind and "dissolve time." (That comes in handy when you are underwater for over twenty minutes holding your breath!)

He stresses acknowledging the reality that we are breathing beings and to experience this reality deeply, in detail. "Breathing is this one constant in life," he says. "Breath coming in and breath going out. We need to explore and experience all the aspects and levels of this amazing process: physiological, emotional, energetic, spiritual."

"Breathwork is a way to come home to yourself, to challenge yourself. It's a way to apply elite concepts to our ordinary activities, a way to rewire the nervous system and to change the way that the brain thinks."

Stig sees breathwork as a way to "really meet yourself and what you are made of; a way to practice self-love and to embrace your life, and yourself, exactly as you are." And it is also a way to "redefine who we are and what is possible."

"When you expand your breathing," he says, "you begin to have bigger thoughts, aspirations, and goals." And in his experience, when we increase our consciousness of breathing, we awaken an entirely new level of consciousness.

He relates breathing to connection and communication between mind and body, conscious and subconscious, and neurons in the brain; he is also passionate about connecting and communicating with nature. He says it's necessary to wake up our symbiotic relationship with the planet, the trees and animals, the streams and rivers—and he has learned that breathing is a way to do that.

He teaches people to mediate, to open and consciously expand out into the world, out into the cosmos, and then to zoom back in on themselves, their bodies, and to use that spiritual energy to charge their batteries. When so-called miracles or superhuman feats occur, he believes it's just nature doing its part.

Stig teaches people to breathe in consciously through their nose. He says, "This is how we tell our brain that we are breathing." He adds: "When you breathe in, imagine you are breathing in the beautiful fragrance of your favorite flower." He also teaches many *pranayama* techniques, such as *ujjayi* (also called "Ocean Breath" and "resistance breathing"). This is done by tightening your throat to produce an internal sound. (Pranayama is the Hindu science of breath.)

Another is *kapalabhati,* in which you draw the belly in forcefully as you exhale, with arms in the air. *Bhastrika,* also called "Warrior Breath," builds on kapalabhati. You raise your arms into the air with the inhale and pull them down forcefully into the lower ribs while shouting "*hah*" from the belly with each exhale.

Stig advises us to practice Breath Awareness and Conscious Breathing throughout the day: when you are on the subway, in the car, while checking your email. He recommends 50 percent water work (breath holding underwater) and 50 percent breathwork (breathing exercises). He is quick to remind us to never do underwater work alone; always use a partner.

Breathwork and PTSD

One of the reasons I love Stig so much is that he is sincerely devoted to helping people with PTSD. When he has the time, he donates his services to veterans and others. He has been known to reserve a block of beautiful hotel rooms; to pay for food, lodging, and even transportation—out of his own pocket—to help people with serious PTSD and train them for free.

His approach is unique. He calls it "underwater meditation," and of course it involves the practice of breath holding. He says: "Breath holding underwater means you can't cheat. You can't fake it!" He sees it as a way to challenge yourself, and in the process, come home to yourself. He encourages people to look at their trauma in a different way, as a challenge to be the best that you can be.

He is honest and direct, and he coaches his clients to be the same. "You have to take responsibility for yourself, for your thoughts and feelings, and stop paying the medical system to keep you sick!"

He says the first step out of the trauma and the drama is to change your focus. "The more you think about it, the more you experience it. Change the way you look at it. If you change your story, you will change your future. Tell yourself you are happy.

Decide to be better, starting right now. No need to focus on trauma: focus on breathing."

Breathwork teaches us to recognize and take advantage of opportunities when they arise. It allows us to focus on and take advantage of internal positive resources and natural abilities that we all have. He starts by telling his students to, "Put everything into each breath: consciousness, passion, enthusiasm, focus, determination, love, and the pain . . . And be willing to go beyond."

Based on my own experience and what I've learned from Stig, I've summarized how the practice of breathwork and breath holding can help with PTSD: when you hold your breath or hyperventilate for a long time, you give yourself an opportunity to bring up and deal with some very strong emotions and urges: fear, anxiety, doubt, and negative and limiting thoughts. By relaxing into these emotions and getting comfortable with them, you are working through your stress and dissolving your anxiety. By bringing up these feelings and natural reactions and working through them voluntarily, you find that you can handle them when they come up in everyday life.

You may not be suffering from PTSD, but the ability to "relax on demand" and to overcome or eliminate stress and anxiety, to conquer fear and negativity, is good for everyone. The self-control and self-confidence that breath mastery brings helps full-time parents and cab drivers, athletes and therapists, surgeons and advertising executives, police and schoolteachers. It helps disabled people, children, and anyone who is ill.

One of the core techniques that Stig recommends and encourages everyone to practice is the simple one-to-two ratio. That means the exhale is twice as long as the inhale. If you inhale for a count of two, exhale for a count of four. If you inhale for a count of four, exhale for a count of eight.

Pick an easy count for the inhale, and then breathe out for twice as long. It's very simple. Focus, and adjust the count as you go, maybe faster or longer. Just make sure that the exhale is twice as long as the inhale. Practice it now and do it for a few minutes throughout your day.

The Art of Breath Holding

Breath holding is an advanced practice to be sure, even though most of us as kids had breath-holding contests and were probably tempted to see how long we could stay underwater.

The therapeutic value of breath holding is extraordinary in many ways. When you hold your breath for an extended length of time, you find yourself dealing with very powerful feelings and sensations, reactions and urges—biological, chemical, emotional, psychological. In the practice of exploring these reactions, learning to relax into them, or to tolerate them, real breakthroughs and permanent healing can occur very quickly. The internal forces that take over despite our conscious will or intention can be humbling, and they can be valuable in terms of overcoming things we mistakenly believe are out of our control.

One tiny piece of advice in breath holding is to hold your breath as long as you can, at least to the point where your diaphragm begins to flutter or spasm, and then hold it for just a moment or two more. Research shows that your brain gets flooded with about 300 percent more blood for about thirty minutes after a long breath hold. It seems to be your brain's way of compensating or balancing out after the emergency—the lack of oxygen—that you created with the breath holding.

There are many ways to hold your breath. For example, you can hold your breath in or you can hold your breath out. You can hold your breath after pulling in a full inhale, or you can hold your breath after a blowing out a complete exhale. And you can also hold your breath at some midpoint, a neutral point in the breathing cycle. You can hold your breath by closing your mouth and pinching your nose, by locking your throat, by using your chest or abdominal muscles, or by controlling your diaphragm. You can hold the breath using a single muscle or a muscle group, or you can spread the workload over all the muscles in the system. You can even learn to hold your breath without using any muscular effort at all.

The breath holding we are talking about here is not for free diving. That is a form of underwater diving that relies on a diver's ability to hold his or her breath until resurfacing rather than relying on breathing apparatus such as scuba gear. If you are interested in free diving, I suggest you train with a pro like Stig Severinsen.

❋ BREATHE NOW: HOW TO HOLD YOUR BREATH

Hold it. How do you do that? What muscles do you use? What do you feel when you hold your breath? Where do you feel it? How long can you hold your breath?

I suggest that you practice breath holding in conjunction with relaxation. Relax everything you can as much as you can while you are holding your breath. Don't use any unnecessary effort or muscular activity.

If you are serious about exploring breath holding, I suggest that you organize your practice. Don't approach it in a haphazard or casual way. Plan to practice for several weeks while sitting at rest, and keep a journal to track your progress.

There are three important keys to this practice:

1. Practice holding your breath out, that is, after your exhale. Take in a normal breath, let it out, then don't breathe in. Hold your breath

at that point. Use a watch or a clock and start your practice by taking these three readings:

> Note when you feel the first clear yet subtle urge to breathe. Mark that time. We call it a "comfortable pause."

> Note when you feel a strong yet manageable urge to breathe. Mark the time. We call it a "controlled pause."

> Hold your breath until the urge to breathe is practically uncontrollable. Mark that time. We call it a "maximum pause."

When you practice, you will be working with the first reading: the comfortable pause after the exhale. That is the pause you want to extend: breath holding after the exhale. In other words, you are postponing the inhale.

2. When you have finished the pause, you should be able to simply resume normal breathing. If you have to take a recovery breath, it means you have gone beyond the comfortable pause. If you have to take in a deep inhale to catch your breath, it means you are not working with that first reading. Practice more awareness. Tune in to your subtle feelings and sensations. Approach the practice more gently. Practice breath holding with some free breathing time between each attempt. Practice for ten or twenty minutes, two or three times a day.

3. Lengthen your comfortable pause by just two or three seconds every two or three days. The idea is to very gradually train yourself and your system to comfortably tolerate higher levels of CO_2. That means you are relaxing into the feelings of air hunger, gradually learning to

tolerate them. Forcing yourself to temporarily override or fight the urge to breathe will bring very few long-term benefits.

Now and then, check the time of your maximum pause. You will find that it has automatically increased significantly. And if you test yourself after taking in a deep inhale, which is what most people do, you may be amazed at your newfound natural ability!

Some breathwork exercises or techniques call for holding the breath in after the inhale. When practicing breath holding at that point, try not to lock up your throat and create back pressure: use an "open hold" or a floating pause. That means keep your throat open and relaxed. If a tiny bit of air escapes, then pull it back in. Give yourself the sense that you are hovering there. That is an open hold, a floating pause.

The same practice can be applied to breath holding at the empty point, after a full exhale. Keep your throat open, and if a tiny bit of air comes in, then immediately send it back out; if a small bit of air leaks in, blow it back out. In this way you are practicing an open hold.

Another practice is to continue to breathe in mentally once you have reached the physical limit of the inhale. It is similar to the open hold technique, but instead of allowing a bit of air to escape and then pulling it back in, you continue to lean in the direction of inhaling more. Give yourself the sense that you are continuing to inhale even though no more air is coming in.

You can practice the same thing after the exhale. Once you have emptied yourself completely, remain open and continue the intention to exhale. Even though no more air is coming out, you have the sense of continuing to exhale. From the outside, or on the surface, it looks and seems as if you are holding your breath, and in a way you are, but the inhale or exhale is actually continuing on the inside, on the level of intention and energy.

Breath holding can also be combined with other things such as meditation, visualization, energy work, various postures, movements, or physical exercises.

In this section I've described breath holding as an exercise in awareness, relaxation, and breath control. If you are interested in exploring it more deeply—for extreme sports, for example—I recommend studying with someone like Stig Severinsen who teaches advanced hypoxic training.

The Buteyko Method: Asthma, Allergies, and More

The Buteyko Method will help with asthma, allergies, hypertension, heart disease, immune deficiency, and cancer.

When I first visited Russia in 1990, it was impossible to mention breathing without someone mentioning Konstantin Buteyko. He was a legend then and remains one posthumously.

When I learned about his method, I began calling mine the "non-Buteyko method," because it seemed that we had completely opposite beliefs and approaches. He said that people breathe too much, and I said that people didn't breathe enough!

In fact, I even joked that only in the Soviet Union could such a method even evolve. Imagine teaching people not to breathe, that deep breathing was bad! Many of his patients or students who came to my seminars seemed afraid to breathe fully, freely, or deeply. This struck a cultural nerve in me, because I came from the land of the free, where we were encouraged to breathe as much as we wanted, even too much if that's what we liked. I thought he was crazy.

But you can't argue with success, and the fact is, the Buteyko Method, especially for asthma sufferers, is extremely effective. I have integrated many of his ideas and methods into my own work over the years, and I suggest that anyone interested in a drug-free approach to healing asthma look into it.

Buteyko was born in 1923 in Ukraine. He entered the university to study engineering, but World War II changed his plans, and he ended up in the army. He was a driver and repaired cars and trucks, but he soon realized that he was meant to repair human bodies. He wanted to heal people, so when the war ended he went to medical school. He graduated with high honors, and was assigned to a very prestigious hospital in Moscow.

Buteyko suffered for many years with a severe case of high blood pressure, and despite access to the best drugs and medical treatments, his condition only worsened. He also suffered from what he called chronic heavy breathing, and he attributed it, as the medical profession did, to his condition.

But one evening, following what he described as a flash of light, he got the idea that his heavy breathing, rather than being the result of his disease, was actually the cause of it. He began to experiment with shallow breathing and breath holding, and ultimately healed his hypertension.

When I met him and asked him how he would summarize his teachings, he said: "Deep breathing is death!" He said carbon dioxide was a vasodilator, and that deep breathing eliminates too much CO_2. This in turn causes vasoconstriction throughout the system, including bronchial vessels, blood vessels, intestines, and so on, which results in all kinds of medical problems.

In fact, he said, asthma is not a disease at all: it is the body's way of trying to preserve carbon dioxide. He said that people with asthma feel as if they need to breathe more, but in fact, they need to breathe less. And that is the basis of his method.

The Buteyko Method is not only a great self-treatment for asthma, it is very useful training if you are an athlete. Here is what I took away from my meetings with him many years ago:

1. Never, ever breathe through your mouth. Do whatever you must to break the habit of mouth breathing.

2. Practice very shallow and quiet nose breaths with lots of long pauses.

3. A healthy person sitting at rest should be able to tolerate a comfortable pause after a normal exhale, for a minimum of thirty to forty-five seconds. To test yourself, simply take in a normal inhale and a normal exhale, then close your mouth, pinch your nose, and don't breathe in. Measure the time before you have to breathe in again, and practice gradually increasing that time.

4. Practice controlled pauses after the exhale, very gradually (over a period of weeks) increasing the length of the pause until you reach a comfortable pause of forty-five or even sixty seconds.

5. If you have to take in a deep breath or two after the pause, you're cheating. You should be able to resume normal breathing without taking a recovery breath. If you have an urge to take in a deep breath after the hold, then fight the urge and take little breaths slowly until you recover.

6. Do mild exercises while breath holding, for example walk-
    ing with your arms above your head and counting your
    footsteps—gradually increasing the number of footsteps you
    can take during the pause.

7. The key is to gently and gradually increase your tolerance of
    the feelings of air hunger and gently control the emotions
    triggered by them.

How to Detox with Breathwork

With every exhale, you are already automatically releasing toxins and
metabolic waste from your system. Nature sees to it that it happens.
However, you can increase the detoxing effect, improve circulation,
and support digestion by combining "kapalabhati pranayama" and
"paradoxical breathing" or "reverse respiration."

    By putting these two breathing exercises together, you get a sense
of stirring, loosening, or shaking everything up with the rapid breathing, then you use the long, slow paradoxical inhale and exaggerated
exhale to squeeze out everything that you brought up.

❋ BREATHE NOW: CONSCIOUS DETOX PRACTICE

Breathing in and out through the nose, do a minute or so of kapalabhati pranayama. This means breathing sharp, rapid breaths using
your abdominal muscles, focusing on the exhales, and allowing the
inhales to be passive or reflexive. Follow this exercise with one or two
long slow paradoxical breaths—drawing the diaphragm up and pulling
in on your belly button and abdomen while you inhale. (With practice,

you can also pull up on the perineum, the area between the anus and the posterior part of the external genitalia.)

As you are inhaling through your nose, imagine drawing waste products up out of your muscles, tissues, organs, and cells. And here is the key: continue to draw up on the diaphragm and pull the belly in even more as you exhale, squeezing out all the breath through your mouth— every last bit. When you are done, simply relax everything. A passive or neutral inhale will automatically occur. Do another minute or so of rapid kapalabhati breathing, and then another couple of long slow paradoxical breaths: try to feel a subtle upward tug throughout your body, starting all the way down in your feet or lower legs as you are breathing in.

Draw the breath all the way up through your torso and up to your throat, and then release the breath through an open mouth while you continue to draw the diaphragm up even higher, while you continue to pull in on the belly even more. Squeeze every last bit of air out, and with it, all the toxins you sucked up out of your muscles, tissues, and cells.

When you have squeezed out all the breath, just relax and let everything go. Allow your breath and body to return to a neutral state, and then do another minute or so of kapalabhati. Alternate back and forth between the rapid kapalabhati breathing and the paradoxical breaths.

Here's another exercise you can do to help release toxins from your system. Take in a breath and hold it in. Then play with the breath as if it is a ball of air that you can move up and down between your chest to your belly, puffing your chest up and then popping your belly out. Move that ball of breath up and down between your lower belly and upper chest.

After some time, release the breath and empty yourself. Then do it again. Take in a breath, lock it into your system with your throat, and bounce and move that ball of air up and down and around in your upper body: sucking the belly in and puffing your chest out, then compressing your chest and popping the belly out. After some time, relax and release the air.

The Nose Knows!

The question that comes up most often at just about every seminar, workshop, or training is: "Should I breathe through my nose or my mouth?"

The nose is meant to be breathed through. Nature designed it for that purpose. It has hairs that filter dust and mucus membranes that trap microscopic particles. It conditions the air, warming or cooling it, depending on what is needed. When we breathe through our nose, we produce more nitrogen oxide, which has antibacterial, antiviral, and anti-fungal properties. And like carbon dioxide, nitrogen oxide is also a vaso-dilator. The nose also has turbinate structures that spiral the air on the way to the lungs. Hmmm . . . why do you think nature would do that?

Breathing through the nose helps us to fine tune our awareness and our sense of subtle energies. And yet the mouth is more flexible: we can shape the stream of breath and play with sound when we breathe through the mouth. It allows more creative possibilities. And of course, you can't laugh or cry or yawn through your nose. You can't express or release powerful emotions through your nose.

Many people cannot breathe through their mouth without trig-gering stress, without activating the sympathetic nervous system or the fight-or-flight response. If you get dizzy or feel uncomfortable when you breathe through your mouth, you may want to fix that. Learn to breathe through your mouth with comfort, pleasure and ease, and to relax and sense subtle energies while breathing through your mouth.

With that ability, you can use breathwork for emotional clearing and spiritual purification. Imagine a house that has not been cleaned in years. Nose breathing would be like dusting the window sills or polishing the silverware. You wouldn't start that way. First you'd sweep or even shovel out all the big, heavy garbage. That's mouth breathing. We will explore when to use nose breathing and when to use mouth breathing in more detail in the Twenty-One-Day Breath Mastery Challenge in Chapter 6.

Yawning Your Way to Better Health

Yawning is a natural breathing technique that will improve your overall health and well-being. It energizes you while also triggering the relaxation response. It helps with sleep, mood, and anxiety, and it discharges stress and tension.

Everywhere I go I encourage people to yawn. Why? Because it's good for you and it feels good too. Yawning is one of those very natural reflexes, and not just among humans. All mammals yawn, as well as birds and reptiles. And although we tend to associate yawning with being tired or bored, there is far more to it than that.

Animals often yawn before they attack, and they yawn when the fight is over. Have you noticed how often dogs and cats yawn and stretch, even after lying for only a few minutes? Yawning has to do with energy, balancing the nervous system, releasing toxins, and more. One of the most interesting things about yawning, and we all know this, is that whenever one person in a group yawns, someone else also does. In fact, just talking about yawning in a group will result in someone yawning.

We know that yawning is contagious, and science is finally beginning to take a more serious look at this phenomenon. Did you know that sociopaths don't share the tendency to yawn when others do? The less empathy a person has, the less likely he or she is to catch a yawn.

Yawning is a very natural and healthy phenomenon. It's actually a vital breathing reflex, but consider the social programming around it. We've been taught to think or feel that it is rude or impolite, even insulting or offensive! Besides attracting attention, there is often a perceived message of boredom, or that the yawner is not interested in what is happening or being said. Cultural mores about open mouths and human noises deem that they are not acceptable in "polite society." All this causes people to suppress something that nature requires us to do.

I imagine a young schoolboy in the back of a classroom allowing a big yawn, surrendering totally to it while the teacher is lecturing or writing something on the blackboard. I imagine this juicy, yummy, luxurious, full-body yawn taking over the child. With the yawn comes the natural urge to stretch and to breathe and to make sounds . . . It's a beautiful moment of natural healthy pleasure and aliveness.

But yawning attracts attention, which sometimes can be negative and punitive. As a result, the child is taught in no uncertain terms to keep that movement of life energy, of that natural spirit, to himself.

In her poem "Wild Geese," poet Mary Oliver says you need to "let the soft animal of your body love what it loves."[7] She may not have been referring to yawning, but that's exactly what it feels like when we allow a full-body yawn to take over our being.

Now imagine you are a counselor or a therapist, and someone is telling you his or her problems: "My dog died." "My teenage son is on drugs." "I lost my job." "My marriage is falling apart." And right then you feel an urge to yawn. What kind of reaction can you expect if you surrender to that urge? "Am I boring you?" "Are you tired?" "Aren't you listening to me?" "Don't you care about me or my problems?" "How dare you yawn right now!"

Would you as a counselor or a therapist allow yourself to yawn in that situation? (All the ones that I have trained certainly would, and not only that, they would encourage their clients and patients to do the same.)

Yawning is a perfectly natural way to integrate, process, and shift energy. It's nature's way of connecting you with your energy, body, and feelings. Yawning allows us to open and connect to another's feelings, to awaken and connect with others on a subtle energetic level. It allows you to touch your own spirit, to open to the flow of the universal life force on a very deep level and in a very practical way.

When we yawn we clear and release subtle energetic blocks in our system, allowing us to feel more fully and deeply into what is happening, into what is being experienced. It allows us to be totally present to ourselves and the ones we are with.

The yawning reflex lights up the same part of our brain that is associated with empathy, bonding, play, and creativity. So please let that soft animal of your body, or that little boy or little girl in you, yawn to his or her heart's content!

If you are like most people, you probably have a lot of incomplete yawns trapped inside of you, aching to come out. Admit it: you have suppressed or blocked or inhibited many yawns throughout your life. So much so that I would wager even when you are alone you probably automatically suppress some portion of the yawn out of habit.

Maybe one reason yawning seems contagious is that it communicates acceptability, it is like giving someone else permission. Subconsciously we think: "Oh, you mean it's okay to yawn here? Good! Because I need it too." Science is now telling us it is a good idea to yawn and to yawn often.

What happens in a dog or cat's jaw, spine, pelvis, and limbs when they yawn? The jaw opens wide, the spine arches and curls. They also stretch their front and back legs as if doing yoga! You need to do that too. When was the last time you really let yourself yawn? Unashamed. Uninhibited. Without any embarrassment or self-consciousness. When was the last time you allowed yourself to enjoy a full total-body yawn? What if yawning is to your energy body what showering is to your physical body?

I like to look at how yawning is similar to other human experiences in terms of the forces and dynamics at work. Think about it: you can trigger a yawn, and you can block or suppress a yawn. But when it's happening, it's very hard to get out of the way of it.

The important words here are "it is happening." You are not "doing" the yawn. You can do something to trigger it, to bring it on, and you can do something to block it or suppress it, but once it's happening, it is happening. You are not doing it. It is something that takes over your body, your being.

What else is like that? How about an orgasm? You can trigger it and you can suppress it, but once it is happening, once it takes over, it is awfully difficult to get out of the way of it! Guess what? Learning to welcome and allow yawning, learning to deliberately enjoy full-body yawns throughout the day, will improve your sex life at night. (But only if you have a belly button!)

Another example of a human experience when similar forces and dynamics are at work is when it comes to emotions. They are contagious. You can trigger an emotion—in yourself or in others—and you can suppress an emotion. But when it is happening, there's no getting out of the way of it. Emotions, when they come up, take over your body-mind system.

Learning to breathe and relax through a yawn helps us to breathe and relax with our emotions; it enables us to channel energy in a more conscious, healthy, and creative way. The unique yawning exercises at the end of this chapter will not only open and expand your breathing capacity, they will help you open to your emotions more fully, to honor and embrace them, but not be so pushed or pulled or controlled by them.

The next exercise combines what I call basic and advanced yawning. I am going to ask you to play with your yawn and to experiment with the yawning reflex. You will be giving yourself big, expansive inhales and luxurious sighs of relief during the yawn. And you will be practicing "connected breathing," spinning the breath like a wheel while you yawn.

Before we get into the practice, I'd like to point out how yawning is just like any other natural urge or reflex—like eating, sleeping, or using the toilet—and yet very different. For example, when you're eating, you don't wait until you are starving to death before you feed yourself. You don't wait until you are exhausted and falling off your feet before you give yourself a rest. And you don't wait until your body is screaming and desperate to relieve itself before you allow it. You do these things on purpose and on a regular basis, often even before you really have to or need to.

We have rituals built into our lives that allow us to do these things often. And yet when it comes to yawning, when do you yawn? You probably only do so when and if your body actually demands it, forces you to do it. And then what do you do? You probably suppress it, either partially or completely.

The point is: don't wait until your body demands yawning. Create daily yawning rituals. Yawn on purpose. Do it often. Do it regularly. Anyone can trigger a yawn. As you breathe in, open your mouth, wiggle your jaw, do something with the back of your throat and trigger the yawning reflex.

Do it now. Do it more than once. Stretch while you yawn. Make a pleasant, soothing sound when you yawn. Yawn till your eyes water. Forget about what people think. Forget about what you think! Forget about how you look. Wherever you are right now, put this book down and give yourself a big juicy, luxurious full-body yawn. Indulge yourself. Go for it! Do it again. Make noise.

How do you feel?

If you cannot allow yourself to experience a full-body yawn, what does that say about all the other areas of your life where you don't let yourself be natural? Do your concerns about what other people will think or say, or how they will react, stop you from listening to your body, to your heart, to your nature?

How often and in how many ways are you inhibiting your own natural energies, your creativity, your love, your truth, your spirit? Stop it! Just stop it! Give yourself (and others) permission to be fully human. When we don't let ourselves and each other be human, we force ourselves and each other to be fake.

The children among us and around us are modeling our behavior; they are consciously and unconsciously adopting our habits and patterns. We need to provide them with an honest example of what is truly natural. Get over your social, family, religious, or cultural programming. Let yourself yawn. Make yourself yawn. Encourage others to get over their stuff about it too.

Yawning is a powerful neural-enhancing tool. In fact, it has been called one of the best-kept secrets of neuroscience. Yawning is associated with the precuneus, a tiny structure hidden within the folds of the parietal lobe, and it appears to play a central role in consciousness, self-reflection, and memory retrieval. The precuneus is associated with the mirror neuron system in the brain. Yawning evokes a unique neural response in the part of the brain involved in social awareness and feelings of empathy. Deliberate yawning can strengthen this important part of the brain and this capacity in us.

Yawning increases when we are tired, and it may be one way our body tells us we need to rest. On the other hand, exposure to light also makes us yawn, which means it's part of the process of waking up. Yawning relaxes us, but it also brings on a state of increased cognitive awareness: it can make us more alert. It helps us become more introspective and self-aware. Yawning is a part of the parasympathetic response—rest and digest mode. It also plays a part in regulating our temperature and metabolism.

You can use yawning to ward off the effects of jet lag and to ease the uncomfortable effects of high altitudes. Athletes use it before performing. Even fish yawn when changing activities! Many neurochemicals are involved in yawning, including dopamine, which activates oxytocin, the neurotransmitter that regulates sensuality and pleasure, as well as bonding in relationships, which means yawning can enhance intimacy. Other neurochemicals associated with yawning include ACTH, MSH, GABA, nitric oxide, serotonin, glutamate, sex hormones, and more. It is believed that yawning also cools off the brain. In fact, neuroscientists can find no other single activity that has so many benefits and influences so many brain functions at once.

What more do I have to say to get you to yawn? What do I have to do to convince you that you need to yawn more? Deliberately trigger a yawn before you do something important, and then yawn after you finish it. Yawn from time to time during tests, tasks, activities, interactions, performances, presentations, and meditation. And yawn whenever you feel anxious, angry, or afraid, tired or wired. You owe it to yourself to enjoy this natural neurological treat. So what are you waiting for? Let's practice right now.

❋ BREATHE NOW: YAWNING 101

Don't close or cover your mouth when you yawn. Look up. Let your jaw fall open.

Follow the urge to stretch when you yawn. Lymph glands in your neck, throat, and armpits are part of your immune system. When you yawn and stretch, you naturally squeeze and activate these vital glands.

Think of dogs or cats: what happens in their jaw, neck, spine, hips, pelvis, and limbs when they yawn? Let that happen in you. Don't just yawn once. Yawn again and again. Yawn until your eyes water. Getting your eyes to water is a very important part of a full natural yawn.

How do you feel?

❋ BREATHE NOW: ADVANCED YAWNING 301

I joke at my seminars that I don't often teach advanced yawning on the first date, and I have never taught it in a book before, but I will assume that you are an advanced being and ready for advanced yawning. Welcome to Yawning 301!

Give yourself a full, total-body yawn as described above. But now bring conscious connected breathing into it. Don't freeze the breath when you yawn. Don't hold your breath when the yawning reflex takes over. Breathe in and out during the yawn.

When you yawn, notice that it produces a special opening in your throat, and it gives your breath a soft, round, open sound. Breathe in and out continuously through that natural opening that the yawn produces. Next, trigger the yawning reflex, and during the yawn, deliberately give yourself big, expansive inhales and big sighs of relief.

The idea is to do connected breathing—also called continuous breathing—during the yawn: give yourself quick, smooth panting breaths, in and out, in and out—like a happy dog! Get that wheel of breath spinning when the yawn is happening.

This technique is at the cutting edge of breathwork today. People who have mastered this simple technique report that they feel physically, emotionally, and psychologically better after a few minutes of this practice. It may be awhile before we know all the medical and scientific benefits of this breathwork technique, so don't wait—be your own scientist. Start practicing it now. Practice it every day. Make this the new way that you yawn.

What if I told you that small elite teams of warriors and some of the top athletic teams around the world are beginning to yawn and breathe together in this way? Now imagine that you or your team stumbled upon something simple and basic and easy, that happens to give you or your team a tremendous advantage over the enemy or the competition. Would you share your practice? Or would you keep it a secret? Yawning is serious business. It's time you started having fun with it!

Here's my secret formula for practicing advanced yawning: 10 + 10 + (10 X 2). That's ten minutes in the morning, ten minutes at night, and ten times during the day for two minutes. In fact, this formula can be applied to any of the breathing techniques, exercises, or meditations in this book. Practicing according to this formula may be the best way to integrate breathwork into your everyday life, and to master any technique or exercise.

Everyday Breathing

I end this chapter (and chapters 3 and 4) with a set of simple yet effective breathing practices for common situations and problems that relate to the body (or mind or spirit). By focusing on your breath and breathing consciously at certain times and in certain situations, you can turn ordinary moments into priceless opportunities to cultivate greater health and well-being, and more peace, power, and presence.

Wake Up

If you get groggy, feel tired, but still have work to do, here's a Sufi technique that will help. (By the way, the Sufis—Muslim mystics—have lots of great meditations and exercises, combining breath with thought, prayer, movement, and sound.)

Give yourself two to four short, quick powerful inhales through the nose, and then blow the breath out through pursed lips. Do that for two minutes, and see if you are not buzzing with energy and aliveness. Shoot these short quick breaths into your chest through the nose, and then release the breath out your mouth through pursed lips. We call this the "Sniff and Pooh Breath" because of the sound you make when inhaling through the nose and when blowing out through pursed lips.

Sniff . . . Sniff . . . Sniff . . . Poooh! Sniff . . . Sniff . . . Sniff . . . Poooh! Sniff . . . Sniff . . . Sniff . . . Poooh! Sniff . . . Sniff . . . Sniff . . . Poooh!

Don't laugh! Or laugh if you want to, but try it. Do it now. And do it again. Play with it. Experiment.

Getting Out of Bed

Charge the body by deeply stretching into the inhale and stretching as you sigh the breath out. Do this three times.

Charge the mind by inhaling for a count of five and exhaling for a count of five.

Charge the heart by focusing the breath in the heart area, and imagine that on the inhale you are breathing in compassion for yourself, and on the exhale you are expressing gratitude for a brand-new day.

Shower

Tune in to your breath as you turn on the tap, and watch how the breath changes as you experience the warm water washing over you. Meet the feelings with the breath. Breathe and open and relax into the feelings, as you would the caressing touch of your beloved.

End your shower by turning on the cold water. Meet the feelings with your breath. Practice breathing in and out quickly and smoothly. Deliberately relax your body and integrate the stimulating feelings of cold water. When you are done, breathe vigorously as you dry yourself off. Take a couple of long, lovely sighs of relief to end the ritual.

Traffic

Stopping at a red light is a good opportunity to relax and do so some cleansing breaths, or use the time just to tune in to your body and your breathing. If you are stuck in traffic, loosen your grip on the wheel. Check your shoulders and your posture. Scan your body, bringing awareness and breath to any places where you find you are holding tension. Breathe as you wiggle and relax your jaw, your neck, and your shoulders.

As soon as you notice any contractions anywhere in your body, return to the breath. Use your breathing to relax and release the tension. You can actually choose to enjoy being stuck in traffic! Turn on a toe-tapping, hand-clapping song, and then breathe in rhythm to the music. Consider how being stuck in traffic compares to what some people have to bear on a daily basis. Shift your focus.

Deliberately generate gratitude and conjure up appreciation. Consciously enjoy the feeling of expansion on the inhale and deliberately enjoy the feeling of relaxation on the exhale. Strengthen that part of you that has the ability to generate comfort and pleasure at will. And remind yourself that life is good.

Treadmill

When you are on the treadmill at the gym, breathe in rhythm to your footsteps. Use the time to work your way through the body, breathing into every part or place you are conscious of. Be conscious of unnecessary tension or effort. Relax any muscles you don't need to maintain your pace and form.

You can also practice breathing into your chakras, repeating an affirmation, mantra, or power statement as you turn your attention and move through each one. (A chakra is a point of subtle energy described in yoga texts. Our body has seven of them, and it is said that the energy in our chakras spins like a wheel. We will discuss them in more detail in the section on Binnie Dansby and Source Process, Letting Go of Life-Limiting Thoughts.)

Headache

Breathe gently into the epicenter of the pain, using your breath to move all your attention into the pain. Then exhale softly and deeply, relaxing the muscles or the area around the pain and tension. Look for details. Is there a shape to the pain? Does it have borders? Does it have a texture? Does it have a temperature?

This isn't about analysis, it's about feeling. Use your breath to bring energy, relaxation, and awareness to the pain. Do this for a few minutes and watch how the sensations move and shift and change. And don't be surprised if the headache passes.

Pain and Fatigue

Most people are very surprised at their ability to release pain and fatigue from their bodies after only a small amount of focus and practice. The same practice we used for a headache can be used for any pain.

The key to breathing in this case is not to make the pain go away, but to find or create comfort in the presence of the pain. If you did or are doing something to cause the pain, then you can do something to stop the pain. But if the pain comes by itself, why not let it go by itself?

The practice is referred to as "butterfly breaths" or "cave breathing." It involves very subtle—almost imperceptible—continuous breathing. You practice a connected breathing rhythm—a wheel of breath—to gently get energy flowing and find or create a space of comfort, even pleasure, in spite of the pain. This means you take tiny breaths, to relax into a very light and subtle breathing pattern, and then wait and watch for an opportunity to take a more expansive breath. It will come by itself at some point. You will sense an expansive breath suddenly rise up from within. When it does, catch it, help it, cooperate with it. Ride it.

You can also learn to "suck" pain and fatigue from your muscles with the inhale and to release it from the body with the exhale. You can use connected breathing for example when running to pump energy into the body—staying ahead of the demand—and you can pump fatigue out from your body with every exhale as you go, not letting it build up.

Use an expanded inhale to "grab" fatigue from the muscles, and invite a more deliberate exhale to "dump" that fatigue out of your body and into the earth as your feet hit the ground. Let gravity help you release the pain and fatigue as you drop your weight and transfer the energy through your feet and into the earth as you run.

If you are involved in an activity that includes repetitive or rhythmic movements, you can coordinate those movements with the breath, finding your own sweet spot to prevent or manage pain or fatigue. Using awareness, you can zero in on a perfect breathing rhythm, rate, and volume to meet and manage your energy demands.

If you are running, you might inhale for two steps and exhale for two; or you might inhale for two and exhale for four. Or you might inhale for four and exhale for two. And you may find yourself intuitively changing it or adjusting your pattern as you go.

Warming and Cooling

Have you noticed that you can use the same breath to warm up your hands as you do to cool off your soup? We know this, but demonstrate it to yourself right now just for fun.

Put the palm of your hand a few inches in front of your mouth and blow with a *hah* sound, as if you want to steam up a mirror. Notice that the breath feels warm. Now purse your lips as if you are going to whistle and blow. Notice that the same breath feels cool.

You can use the breath to warm yourself up (some yogis have mastered this to such an extent that they can sit in winter and melt the snow around them) or cool yourself off, depending on your situation (or time of season).

To warm yourself up: breathe through the nose and quickly pump the breath with your belly and diaphragm (similar to the kapalabhati or "Breath of Fire").

To cool yourself, turn your tongue up toward the roof of your mouth and inhale slowly, feeling the cool sensations under your tongue and in your throat. Consciously draw that breath all the way down to your perineum, and feel it cooling your chest and belly along the way.

Remember, in every case, your consciousness and your intention are the prime creative factors that produce your desired results.

Hangover

The detox breathing techniques we discussed earlier in this chapter will also help with hangovers. Remember to rest, because the less sleep you get, the worse your hangover is.

Remember too that exercise releases endorphins, so it can help you get over a hangover. Oxygen increases the rate at which alcohol toxins are broken down, so fresh outdoor air will add a natural boost to your breathing practice.

Last and most important, don't forget to drink water. It's a universal solution (pun intended).

You can apply specific breathing techniques to address the various hangover signs and symptoms, such as headaches, sleepiness, nausea or queasiness. Breathwork can also address the guilt, shame, depression, or anxiety that may accompany a hangover.

Active breathwork exercises work well because they get your blood pumping and your oxygen flowing. And they work especially well when you combine them with various yoga postures or any twisting or bending movements that force blood into the digestive tract.

Weight Loss

Our lungs are the principal excretory organ for weight loss, and since oxygen plays the primary role in burning fat, breathwork is a no-brainer for weight loss.

When a pound of fat is oxidized, about 20 percent of it turns into water and is eliminated, and the other 80 percent is excreted as CO_2, so breathing is literally the main way we lose weight. The carbon in carbon dioxide is fairly heavy, relatively speaking. In fact, the average person breathes out close to a half pound of it every day without even trying.

Whatever exercise you do, if you simply breathe more deeply, you can add to the fat-burning potential of the exercise. Exaggerating the "squeeze and breathe" exercise is good for weight loss, and "reverse respiration" as well as "hypopressive breathing" (learn more about this technique at the end of this section) can also be done as weight loss exercises. Those same exercises also help to deal with hunger pangs.

The technique I like best is this: inhale, and as you do, suck in your belly and pull up on your perineum as well as everything in your abdomen, just like you do with reverse respiration and hypopressive breathing.

Then as you exhale, suck in the belly even more and pull up even more on everything in the abdomen, as you did for detox breathing. Hold the breath and the tension for a long count (for example, ten seconds).

This is not as complicated as it sounds. Just imagine what you would do if you wanted to pretend that you had a very flat belly and a very thin waist. You would suck everything in and up, right? Well, that's it! Do that while you inhale, exhale, and hold.

Insomnia

This technique is recommended by Dr. Andrew Weil for insomnia: breathe in for a count of four, hold for a count of seven, exhale for a count of eight. Some people find that this exercise keeps them busy, thinking and doing. But it is worth a try, because many people say it works for them.

Another technique for insomnia is to remember the Stig Severinsen mantra: "Relaxation is in the exhalation." Use each exhale to imagine and feel yourself slowing down. Make each exhale like the last "chug" of a train coming to a stop. Feel your muscles relaxing, your body softening with each breath.

The technique I like to use is to inhale gently and release the exhale and "puddle out," meaning totally relax the body as the breath pours out. I imagine myself dropping down . . . settling in . . . The breathing is slow and easy and the focus is on relaxing all the joints and muscles, surrendering to gravity, and creating the sensation of melting with each exhale. Make sure not to disturb the relaxation with the next inhale. Don't use effort or force to breathe in; continue to relax as you inhale.

Hypopressive Breathing

Would you like to activate your sympathetic nervous system, strengthen your core, and increase anaerobic strength? Reduce your waist size and flatten your belly? Raise your metabolism and increase muscle tone in your abdomen and pelvis? Improve your sexual function? Treat or prevent hernias, uterine prolapse, incontinence, and constipation? Then play with hypopressive breathing.

Hypopressive breathing is a Chinese medical breathing exercise that was made popular in physical therapy by Marcel Caufriez in the mid-1980s. Basically this exercise involves holding your breath as you pull up on the perineum and pull in on the belly after a full exhale.

Start by taking in a big inhale and expanding the chest. Then squeeze all the breath out and hold it out.

Now act as if you are inhaling. Expand the chest, but don't actually let any air come in. Pull your belly button in toward your spine and pull up on your perineum.

You will feel your chest expand and get the sense that all your abdominal organs are being sucked up into the chest cavity.

Hold this upward pressure for about ten seconds, then relax and breathe in.

Repeat this for about twenty minutes. If you combine it with various postures and stretches, you'll get all the best benefits of abdominal crunches and other abdominal exercises without any of the risks.

Breathwork for Addiction

Breathwork as an aid in the prevention, treatment, and recovery from substance abuse and drug addiction is proving itself to be extremely effective. It has helped many people to reclaim their lives. In fact, in my experience, it works so fast and so well, it's like cheating! The therapeutic technique of choice is Rebirthing-Breathwork. This practice triggers a heightened feeling of energy and aliveness, and produces a natural high that makes drug use less appealing, and even pointless. Rebirthing-Breathwork, also called Connected Breathing, is described on page 193, and it is the final lesson in the Twenty-One-Day Breath Mastery Challenge.

3

BREATHING TO TRANSFORM YOUR MIND

When the breath wanders, the mind also is unsteady.
But when the breath is calmed, the mind too will be
still, and the yogi achieves long life. Therefore, one should
learn to control the breath.

—SVATMARAMA, *HATHA YOGA PRADIPIKA*

On my first visit to Bolivia, I lectured at the Catholic University in La Paz, and did breathwork sessions at the San Pedro Federal Penitentiary. I was a fan of the Prison Ashram Project started by Ram Dass many years earlier, and Leonard Orr and I had done breathwork in Fort Grant Prison in Arizona. So I was quite used to prison environments, but the culture at the San Pedro prison was very different.

For example, one of the prisoners ran a busy restaurant and a small shop in the courtyard. If you wanted a coffee or a hamburger or a roll of toilet paper, you paid cash in full up front—no exceptions, no compromises. However, if you wanted a bag of dope, you could get that now and pay him next Tuesday!

There were two sides of the prison: one side held between eighty and a hundred men who had money or friends or influence. It was orderly as far as prisons go. However, on the other side of the wall, there were nearly two thousand prisoners. There I saw a half dozen guys packed into a cell the size of my bathroom back home, and they seemed to be wearing the same worn-out clothes they came in with years ago.

I can't imagine what the food was like in that part of the prison. I heard fights and gunshots and screaming from where I was working—the safe, cushy side.

Every day, I walked past hundreds and hundreds of people—family members, I guess—lined up outside the prison gates, mostly in a futile attempt to visit people. Meanwhile, money, drugs, weapons, and who knows what else were pouring into the place through every crack and crevice in the security there.

I spent all my time on the "nice" side where most of the inmates had their own cells, and some of them had their own cell phones. They could lock their cell from the inside, and they had food brought in from the outside. Their girlfriends would bring gifts of all kinds, and they were even allowed to stay overnight. It was almost like a motel.

At the time, a former mayor in Bolivia, who was called Flacco by his friends, was serving a prison sentence. Flacco was extremely depressed. His prison pals were worried about him, and they begged me to help him in some way. So I began to spend time with Flacco in his comfortable two-level prison apartment.

He told me that he was in prison because his political enemies had framed him, but the newspapers said he stole millions of dollars from the government coffers. Whom to believe?

I did get a truly unforgettable lesson from him in the power of toxic self-talk, learning very quickly why he was so depressed. Within five minutes of meeting him, he launched into his story about how he had been betrayed by his closest friends and associates, about how unfair it was that he was sitting in prison while the real criminals were allowed to remain free. He went on about how a group of government officials tried to bribe him, and when he refused, they set him up and took him down. He moped about his wife and children, from whom he had become estranged, and how he knew things about the highest officials in the land that would get him killed if he revealed them. He was paranoid to say the least.

I listened sympathetically at first. But then, no sooner had he finished the long, sad story, he started over and repeated everything to me again; and then again, and again, between coffees, over lunch, and then again at dinner, as if for the first time. I was becoming depressed just listening to him! It was like he had a tape playing over and over in his head, and when he opened his mouth it played out loud. Any attempt to change his looping tune was pointless.

I knew that Conscious Breathing had the power to disrupt the pattern of negative inner dialogue people experience to one degree or another. In his case it was extreme. I couldn't even convince him to get up and move around, or to simply stop talking and try just breathing for a few minutes. It seemed impossible for him to hear anything I said, or do anything I suggested. His mind, like an untrained rottweiler, kept pulling him back onto its familiar depressing track.

With my increased persistency, he finally relented and agreed to give Conscious Breathing a try. It was a struggle for both of us, and getting him to stay with the process for more than a few breaths seemed impossible. So we decided to start with a small target: focus on taking ten full free breaths without stopping to swallow or talk or scratch or stretch. That was it: a mini goal!

After a number of attempts, he finally got there. Then we aimed for twenty, and then thirty. We agreed to do three full minutes of uninterrupted continuous and connected breathing (known as the rebirthing technique, developed by Leonard Orr): active inhales and passive exhales, with no pauses between the inhales and exhales and no pauses between the exhales and the inhales.

After his first three-minute practice, he talked at length about the strange feelings and sensations that the breathing activated in his body. It seemed that the feelings were actually strong enough to distract him from his usual train of negative thoughts. Breathing was trumping his toxic self-talk. He was beginning to get out of his head and into his body. When he completed his second three-minute practice, he had an amazing breakthrough. His eyes lit up, and he began to smile. He proclaimed: "We need to celebrate!" I visited him for the next two weeks and through all that time, he remained in that positive state.

He got onto his phone and called the leader of a famous band from Argentina. The next day, a group of musicians were in the courtyard giving us all a live performance. He laughed and sang and danced while waving handkerchiefs in both hands. It confirmed to me once again the power of Conscious Breathing to interrupt our mental chatter and reverse even the most severe downward, negative spirals.

Letting Go of Life-Limiting Thoughts

Binnie A. Dansby is an inspiring teacher and a gifted therapist, healer, writer, and philosopher. She is among the most experienced breathworkers on the planet and founder of a personal and professional development system called Source Process, which has a host of amazing tools and techniques for empowerment. For over thirty years, she has been guiding people in the healing and release of life long wounds of fear, inadequacy, and limitation.

Her work focuses on how the memories of our time in the womb are held in every cell of our bodies. How our consciousness of society is established and nurtured in the womb, and how the quality of our birth affects the quality or our lives, and in turn shapes the quality of society.

Healing birth trauma is the process of changing life-limiting decisions that we made when we took our first breath. Healing begins in the moment we accept the possibility of change, the possibility of continuing to evolve on all levels of being, just as we did in the womb. Healing the first breath, however, is a process that is not always ecstatic and pain-free.

In fact, the process of growth and evolution is one of pushing beyond our old concepts of comfort and testing new frontiers. We can move to a new and expanded experience of union with our body. It is possible to trust the process of life as a healing process.

In a chat over lunch at a conference last year, Binnie said: "Source Process and breathwork is both a philosophy and a psychospiritual practice that includes the breath as a tool to release physiological and psychological stress. It is possible to eliminate primal trauma and transform the subconscious impression of birth into a gentle, awakening event."

The core purpose of Source Process is to free the breath from the physical constrictions caused by the pain and fear we experienced during our birth and to support the integration of the "archetypal affirmations." The archetypal affirmations are fundamental thought forms that bring up specific life-limiting thoughts in order to release them from our consciousness. They are the healing response to the "archetypal negatives."

The use of conscious, connected breathing together with the use of affirmations is a time-tested method for creating change in awareness and behavior. Uniting these two powerful forces with attentive guidance produces sustainable psychological and physiological results.

Each archetypal affirmation corresponds directly to a specific energy center, or chakra, and the color associated with that center or body system. These are:

First chakra, base of the spine, red: "My body is safe, no matter how I may be feeling. I am the earth; I am creativity."

Second chakra, navel, vibrant orange: "I am surrounded by love and support from all the beings in my life. Everything and everyone in physical form is here to support me in physical form."

Third chakra, solar plexus, yellow: "All of my feelings are safe. I am the one who chooses what to think and how to use my energy."

Fourth chakra, heart, green: "I am the innocent child of a gentle universe. I deserve to experience all of my love and compassion."

Fifth chakra, throat, aquamarine: "I am an expression of love. My expression is welcome."

Sixth chakra, third eye, deep blue: "I am connected in love to all that lives and all that breathes. I am connected to divine intelligence that knows my good."

Seventh chakra, crown, royal purple (a blend of the color red for safety, and the color blue for connection): "I am spirit manifest in beautiful physical form. I am a gift from God to the earth. My love is received."

✳ BREATHE NOW: ARCHETYPAL AFFIRMATION PRACTICE

Tens of thousands of thoughts are generated by our mind every day. The choice we make about what to give attention to is determined by our source beliefs, the archetypal decisions and thoughts that are held at the ground of our being.

We are conscious of some of these deep beliefs and not of others. The breath combined with archetypal affirmations can lift the veil and reveal the false beliefs about life and ourselves that we have been holding on to since birth.

1. Begin breathing gently and fully in a continuous, connected rhythm, and pay attention to the thoughts that are triggered when an archetypal affirmation is introduced. Allow all your thoughts to flow. Don't take any of those thoughts personally.

2. Take a deep breath and choose whether you want to place your attention on an archetypal affirmation or the negative thought that it brings up. Choose your source.

Breathe and know that: *Who I am is not any of my thoughts. Who I am is consciousness that is cocreating and choosing in every moment how to use my precious life energy.*

3. Breathe deeply and fully and ask yourself: "What way of thinking is going to produce a feeling of connection and peace, joy and sat-

isfaction? What thoughts or environment do I consciously choose to nourish with my breath, my life energy, to produce optimum health and well-being? What do I choose to inhale? What do I choose to inspire?"

The word "inspiration" refers to both the breath and to the creative principle. What inspires you becomes the inspiration you are to others. Be aware of the creative impulse arising in you when you breathe consciously. Allow it, and inspiration will expand in you. What inspires you awakens your true being and your true purpose. When you allow yourself to be creative, you awaken the impulse in others. The expression of your true being is an inspiration to everyone.

For more information about Binnie and her work, visit: http://bin nieadansby.com/.

Dr. Stan Grof and Holotropic Breathwork

No book on the modern breathwork movement would be complete without mentioning Dr. Stan Grof and Holotropic Breathwork.

Stan Grof was born in 1931 in Prague, where he received an MD from Charles University and his PhD from the Czech Academy of Sciences. Involved in the earliest days of LSD research, he discovered that breathwork could produce many of the benefits of psychotropic drugs without all the chemical risks. He is one of the founders of transpersonal psychology, and was the founding president of the International Transpersonal Association.

Dr. Grof has introduced the world to a new paradigm in psychotherapy, a new form of psychology that integrates the spiritual and mystical aspects of life, where healing is self-regulated and takes place in the heart. It is a radical innovation, and differs entirely from cognitive, talk-based therapies.

Holotropic Breathwork focuses on a flow, a process, rather than on a goal or outcome. It naturally leads the soul to an experience of our own divinity. People are encouraged to begin a session with faster and somewhat deeper breathing, tying inhalation and exhalation into a continuous circle of breath (very similar to the Rebirthing Breathwork technique). Once in the process, they find their own rhythm and way of breathing.

Holotropic Breathwork can be used to intensify the emotions and physical energies underlying various issues and symptoms, and bring them to conscious experience and full expression. The quality of attention and the attitude toward the experience is more important than the speed and intensity of the breathing. Sessions include loud, provocative, rhythmic music, which varies depending on the stage of the process. The combination of music with faster breathing has a remarkable activating effect on the psyche and consciousness-expanding power. Participants are encouraged to suspend any intellectual activity, which is a way of avoiding the emotional impact.[8]

I have provided a very brief description of Holotropic Breathwork here. Not everyone is a candidate for this kind of work because it can have some intense negative effects in some cases. The best advice I can give you is to read Dr. Grof's book *Holotropic Breathwork,* and visit http://groffoundation.org or www.stanislavgrof.com.

Breathing Away Stress

The subject of stress has made its way into mainstream culture in a big way. Yet for the most part it still goes unrecognized and unaddressed in our everyday life, the debilitating effects taking a toll on body, mind, and spirit.

We suffer a host of physical, emotional, and psychological symptoms caused by stress, but when it comes to doing something about it, we merely treat those symptoms instead of addressing the cause.

In fact, a certain amount of stress is good for us, even necessary. We need it to grow and to build resilience. The key is the way we think about it and react to it. Used properly, channeled wisely, stress can strengthen and inform us.

The Hungarian endocrinologist Hans Selye, who coined the term "stress," said that if he had had a better mastery of the English language, he would have used the term "strain" instead, because that's what he really meant. The confusion around this led to all the talk about the difference between "good" stress and "bad" stress.

For the purpose of this discussion, let's assume that stress is "bad." Let's assume that it has become something we need to fix or manage or reduce or overcome. In that case, let us approach it holistically—as a spirit, mind, and body issue. Approach it with mind intelligence, body intelligence, and heart intelligence. Fortunately, the breath is central to all three of these.

There are ways of breathing that reduce stress and ways that exacerbate and even create it. We will explore some of those breathing patterns now. A general rule of thumb for antistress breathing is "low and slow." That means slow diaphragmatic breathing, preferably at a rate of six to eight breaths per minute, or even slower if it is not in any way a challenge.

Another breathing pattern that is used to relieve stress is to make your exhales longer than your inhales. Deliberately extend or lengthen your exhale as you focus on letting go and relaxing. Quiceting your mind, managing your self-talk, and deliberately engaging in positive internal dialogue, using positive affirmations, can help the process immensely.

One of the best teachers I know when it comes to stress management, prevention, and recovery is not a service member, not an extreme athlete, not a high-level CEO. She is a bright, wise, and gentle physician, an integrated medical practitioner in Johannesburg, South Africa. Her name is Ela Manga, and she is dedicated to bringing mindfulness back into medicine.

Dr. Manga specializes in "energy management" and is writing a book on the subject called *My Energy Codes*. Through this methodology, she supports both individuals and teams in healing the effects of stress and burnout. She teaches her patients, clients, and students the difference between genuine or natural energy, which restores us, and "adrenalized energy," which depletes our life force and creates stress.

In her book, Dr. Manga writes:

> *We are facing a global personal and collective energy crisis. Being busy and exhausted is becoming a shared narrative of modern living. Feeling like wide-eyed zombies is a common collective state. Statistics are revealing that burnout is an alarming and common phenomenon of our times. We can't afford to wait until our health and performance gets compromised before we wake up to the conversation about energy. . . . The nature of modern life demands that we develop new skills to grow and thrive. Energy management is one of those skills.*[9]

Dr. Manga teaches energy management through what she calls the "Five Laws of Energy." She and I have created a unique set of breathing exercises and meditations based on each of these laws.

1. Waves: Energy occurs in waves. The whole of nature pulsates with the rhythmic ebb and flow between a high-energy activated state and a quiet state of relaxation. We see it in the waves of the ocean, the lunar cycle, the seasons, our heartbeat, and of course, our breathing. The very functioning of our cells depends on the oscillation of this energy. This oscillation requires us to create balance in our system. To do that we need to balance our breathing: equalize the inhale, which activates the sympathetic branch of the autonomic nervous system, and the exhale, which activates the parasympathetic branch.

Breathing Practice: Breathe in and out in a one-one pattern. Depending on your skill and comfort level, or the state of energy you find yourself in, that could be inhaling for one second and exhaling for one second; or inhaling for two and exhaling for two; or in four and out four; in eight, out eight, etc.

There is a slight pause between the in-breaths and out-breaths, and between the out-breaths and in-breaths—a very conscious and deliberate moment of transition.

2. Still Point: Movement, growth, and expansion are dependent on these waves and cycles, but also on anchoring us to a center point of balance that is still and calm. It is the eye of the storm. This is the real source of natural energy and creativity that is often felt in the mountains and near the ocean. When we tap into this source of energy and inspiration, we are peaceful, joyful, compassionate, calm, trusting, and connected with our gut feelings and authentic power.

Breathing Practice: That still point is found in the pause midway through the inhale or midway through the exhale. If zero is completely empty, and ten is completely full, then the point you want is five. If you have not done enough breathing training to easily recognize this neutral place, then you can simply pull in a big inhale, then relax and let the exhale go with a sigh of relief. Where the air stops coming out of its own accord should be near that neutral midway point. Hover there. Rest there. Relax there. Meditate there.

3. Three Portals: Natural or authentic energy expresses itself in our system through the physical body, the mind, and the heart. It is essential to understand and support all three energy portals and develop body intelligence, mind intelligence, and heart intelligence.

Breathing Practice: First, imagine breathing into, with, and from the center of your brain (the pineal gland). Focus there as you inhale and exhale (perhaps for one to three breaths). Then breathe into, with, and from your lower belly, the place called the *dan tien* in China or the *hara* in Japan. It is the center of gravity in your body, a couple of inches below your navel, midway front to back (again, for one to three breaths). Last, focus on the center of your heart. Breathe into, with, and from this place (again, for one to three breaths). Repeat this cycle, bringing your awareness to these three points of body, mind, and heart intelligence.

4. Unique: Every living form is a unique expression of creative energy. No single leaf or tree is exactly the same. No one person is the same, so we each have different methods to support and express our energy.

Breathing Practice: Here's where you can get very creative. It's up to you to invent interesting patterns, play with rhythm, speed, volume, focus, sound, and so on. It's a breathing version of contact improvisation dance. The idea is to play, to be creative. A simple example could be breathing to the rhythm of the simple "one, two, cha-cha-cha"; or breathing to the rhythm of a waltz: "one, two, three, one, two, three"; or inhaling a series of small bits of air, then exhaling in a long *ahhh*. There are no rules. You are setting your creative energies loose on the breath. Another game might be to make every breath different from the last, varying each breath so no two are the same. Let comfort and pleasure be your guide.

5.   Moving and Changing: In physics, the law of energy states that energy can be neither created nor destroyed, but just changed from one form to another. Energy is never constant. It is always moving and changing forms. For example, we can transform mental energy into physical energy or physical energy into emotional energy.

Breathing Practice: If you are feeling stressed or anxious, try transforming that emotional or mental energy to physical kinetic energy by lengthening your exhalation. This activates the vagus nerve, which stimulates the parasympathetic nervous system. This is a quick and simple way to "change your state."

Dr. Ela Manga's ABC

Helping people to get comfortable with feelings is another way that Dr. Manga uses breathwork. Making space for feelings ("feeling it rather than feeding it") is a powerful way to create new neural pathways. She has created an energy code called ABC to help her clients:

Awareness: Become aware of what you are experiencing physically, emotionally, mentally, without doing anything about it.

Breathing: Make space for what you are becoming aware of by breathing into it, and allowing it to move.

Conscious Choice: Once you have done A and B, you will be more equipped to consciously respond to a situation and make a choice about it rather than reacting to it in a habitual or counter-productive way.

You can learn more about Dr. Ela Manga by visiting her website: www.drelamanga.com.

Breathwork in the Warrior World

If there's anyplace where one needs awareness, energy, courage, endurance, grace, and power, it's on the battlefield. Soldiers need to be able to manage and control their minds, bodies, and emotions, and breathing is the key to awakening and strengthening them. No matter what kind of a leader you are, you can make use of the breathing techniques that the following warriors have to offer. A victory in the boardroom can sometimes be just as important as a victory on the battlefield.

My friend Leonard Orr once said: "Everyone is following someone. And maybe the person you are following is following you! So maybe what we need to do is stop following and start leading." In a way, we are all called to be leaders.

If you are in a formal leadership position in any field—business, sports, medicine, education, counseling—you will need confidence and courage, you will need to stay calm and perform well under pressure, and breathwork will help you to embody these skills and abilities.

What follows here are the stories and techniques of several masters—individuals who embrace, practice, teach, and lead. They are warriors in the true sense of the word. They have made me a stronger leader, and I am honored to count them as friends, teachers, as well as students.

Brigadier General James Cook, US Army (Retired)

My friend General Cook spent over thirty years in the military. He has a degree in biochemistry and a deep understanding of physiology. He served as an infantryman, Army Airborne Ranger qualified, and he retired as a general in 2012. He was the twentieth Commander of the 91st Training Division, which trains all services for deployment to overseas contingency and humanitarian missions. He is also a free diver and he practices Buddhist meditation. "I go to the ocean to reawaken my creativity and peace," he said.

To appreciate General Cook's foundational balance as a warrior and humanitarian, we must recognize that the source comes from his parents. During the occupation of Japan, his father, a soldier, met his future wife and fell in love; after a lengthy courtship, they married and had James. His father was of Irish and Native American descent, and his mother was of a samurai bloodline. Although James was born in Japan during a very turbulent time, his parents gave him the values and benefits derived from the synergistic union of three beautiful cultures.

During our first breathing session, General Cook was able to access a deep state of energy, confidence, and calmness, which he calls his "center of peaceful feelings."

I once asked him how he uses his breath and what benefits there are to Conscious Breathing. He said: "Breath Awareness is meditation, and meditation is a perfect approach to attention training or concentration training.

"I use breathing to scrub out all the noise and junk from my system. It's like a deep energetic cleansing. I use it in critical moments and also in my day-to-day life, for example, when I need to 'go inside' or block out mental noise and distractions.

"The mind can fabricate a lot of fears," he said, "and it is vital to be able to distinguish between the real and the fabricated—otherwise, when you only have a split second to react, you can do the wrong thing." Breathing keeps us conscious, present, and in touch with reality.

General Cook told me of an experience he had one icy, snowy night on a mock patrol during his Army Ranger training. He basically fell off the side of a mountain! He rolled and tumbled and bounced "ass over teakettle," as they say, more than two hundred feet, in pitch darkness. As it was happening, rather than panic, he accessed his training. He described it as a peaceful calm "that came over me like a blanket"; he felt as if something was guiding him from within.

He managed not only to survive but to do it without breaking a single bone. When he finally came to a crashing halt at the bottom of the mountain, he realized that he was still holding on to his M-16.

Now that's the kind of presence of mind we need in a soldier. No wonder he rose through the ranks to become a general!

"This peace that seems to pass understanding can be hard for the ego to grasp," he said. And then he told me of a funny incident in Iraq, when he decided to join his men on a security convoy one night. It wasn't his responsibility, but he said, "I just wanted to be with my folks. It's all part of leadership." They were all dressed in full body armor and riding in an MRAP (an armored military vehicle specially equipped to withstand roadside bombs).

As they drove, he was breathing, meditating, and practicing situational awareness, settling into that "peaceful inner state." His guys kept looking over at him and asking him if he was okay. He kept saying, "Sure." But finally he said, "Why do you keep asking?" And they answered, "Sir, it's just that you look too damn calm!" That combination of deep inner calmness coupled with energy and alertness is a powerful state, and it is one that he has learned to access through breathing.

On another occasion, he was with the 82nd Airborne on a night-fire exercise in Yakima, Washington. He was leading a team that was calling in large mortar rounds. It was very cold and windy, but his Ranger training had taught him mind over matter: "If you don't mind, it don't matter!"

While breathing and relaxing, he happened to notice an area about a hundred yards away that "looked warmer," and so he directed his team to move over to it. As soon as they took up their position in that new location, a mortar round went off exactly where they had been just a few moments before. No one was hurt, but a piece of shrapnel bounced off a portion of his helmet. He keeps it as a souvenir of his intuition.

General Cook says that breathwork connects us to a sort of internal GPS. "Call it intuition, call it what you like," he says, "but it is real. And all of us can learn to access it by practicing Breath Awareness. Everyone has a shield, or a natural ability to avoid danger," he continued, "by unconscious perception or through intuitive feeling. Breathing meditation awakens and strengthens this ability."

General Cook loves free diving. He once told me: "As soon as I put my face in the water, I'm in the zone!" Breath holding awakens a kind of music in him. It's a state of nonthinking. "We miss all the beauty when we focus only on the technical stuff. It's all about freedom. It's about becoming part of the water, part of the flow."

He is also devoted to serving homeless veterans, and those suffering from PTSD and traumatic brain injury (TBI): "It's all about being kind and listening." One of the first things that he did when he retired was to let his hair grow. In eighteen months, it grew to thirteen inches in length. He had it cut off and donated to Locks of Love, an organization that serves people with cancer or who are undergoing chemotherapy. The man is all heart, and the more he breathes, the bigger his heart gets!

General Cook's favorite practice is Breath Awareness or breath watching, to be performed in conjunction with situational awareness: he uses slow, quiet, paced breathing to keep himself in a relaxed, calm, alert, and energized state. His inhales and exhales remain equal and balanced, smooth, and at ease even under extreme stress.

For more information about General Cook, visit his haiku website: www.zenroadwarrior.com.

Mark Divine: Former Navy SEAL Commander

Commander Mark Divine is truly a high-quality human. He humbly models what it takes to be the best in any field: he's got brains. He's got balls. And most of all, he's got a big heart—the size of Mount Everest!

Commander Divine graduated Basic Underwater Demolition/ SEAL training as Honor Man, which means he was first among the 185 men who started the training and the nineteen who completed it. A successful businessman and devoted family man, he is the author of *The Way of the Seal; 8 Weeks to SEALFIT; Unbeatable Mind;* and his newest, *Kokoro Yoga.* He leads the SEALFIT Training Center in San Diego, California. And he embodies much of what this book is about: he's an ordinary man who learned to use the breath to aid him in achieving extraordinarily high levels of performance and peak flow states.[10]

Mark has developed a model called the Five Mountains. They represent the five areas in life that he believes we all need to master. They are:

1. Physical mountain
2. Emotional mountain
3. Psychological mountain
4. Intuitive/awareness mountain
5. Kokoro, or the spiritual mountain

He also created a program that he calls the 20X Challenge. It is based on forming a belief that you can accomplish twenty times more than you think you are capable of, and then setting about in a systematic way to prove to yourself that it's true. He says: "Our spirit thrives on challenges." He has his students and clients create and attain daily, weekly, monthly, and yearly challenges.

When I asked him to explain how he is able to exhibit such high levels of potential and performance, he said: "It's all about the breath." And he said: "When it comes to breathing, it's all about training. Concepts get you nowhere, training gets you everywhere."

Commander Divine told me that he had a secret weapon when he joined the SEALs, which gave him an advantage over the others: he had already spent several years studying breathing and meditation with a Japanese Zen master.

He noticed that the other SEAL candidates were struggling and falling behind because they had not learned Breath Awareness and breath control, and they had not learned to manage their mental and emotional states. He also realized that: "It's easier to keep up than it is to catch up."

I asked Commander Divine to walk me through his use of the breath before a firefight, during the actual engagement, and after the mission. I asked him what he taught his guys to do when they were in the helicopter on the way to a mission. Here's what he told me:

Practice breath control. His core technique is called Box Breathing. This means to inhale for a count of four; hold for a count of four; exhale for a count of four; and hold for a count of four. (It also could be 5-5-5-5, or 6-6-6-6. The point is to make the duration of the inhales, exhales, and pauses of equal length.)

Practice attention control and arousal control. This is about mental and emotional state management. He makes it clear that this is far more important than just physical or athletic abilities. He talks about feeding the "courage wolf" and starving the "fear wolf." This means that we don't allow any performance-degrading imagery or negative internal dialogue. It means engaging only in positive internal dialogue and visualizing success.

He teaches the use of power statements like "Easy day!" or "I got this!" He said his favorite one—the one that got him through the toughest moments in SEAL training—was "Looking good, feeling good, ought to be in Hollywood!" He points out that repeating it in a singsong way makes it work even better.

"When you hit the ground," he said, "you shift into tactical breathing." That means you drop the breath holding, and just breathe continuously, inhaling four and exhaling four. Breathe in and out the nose, or in the nose and out the mouth.

"Breathing training," he says, "releases us into a higher order of functioning, where our perceiving brain is automatically scanning for danger and opportunities." He has learned that Conscious Breathing allows us to access the full capacity of the brain: not just thinking and planning, but intuition and insights.

When the game is on, when you are in action, involved in accomplishing your mission, it's time for setting and completing "micro goals": identifying the one thing that needs to be done and doing it. Focus on it, complete it, and then move on to the next one thing. "The most important thing together with the breathing," he says, "is mental or emotional management. With practice, the positivity collapses into a silent mantra running in the background as you do what needs to be done."

He summarizes the key priorities in this way: breath control, arousal control, attention control, and goal setting (accomplishing micro goals). "When in doubt," he says, "always come back to the breath." Can you see why I freakin' love this guy?

After the mission, he advises his guys to do "box breathing," alone or together. The focus is on reviewing what went well and what didn't, reframing and letting go of regrets. To help with recovery, he teaches gentle movement or stretching while breathing to "bleed the stress out of the muscles." He also teaches "relaxation breathing," which means the exhales are twice as long as the inhales.

To illustrate the power and value of his breathing training, Mark shared a parachuting experience he had when another jumper lost control and collided with him, causing his chute to collapse in mid-air. He had to cut himself loose. Free falling, with only seven seconds left, he remained perfectly calm and managed to deploy his reserve chute just before hitting the ground. He breathed into a hard but perfect landing at about sixty miles an hour, without suffering any injuries! His first thought was about his team member who had collided with him. Was he okay?

Mark Divine guides people into becoming the best possible versions of themselves. He encourages them to show up at their very best every day, no matter what, and he inspires them to serve others from a place of integrity and excellence. He is a lifelong student of the breath, and he practices what he preaches.

Here is a peek into Mark's daily morning ritual—you would be wise to create something similar for yourself:

When he wakes up, he drinks a glass of water and does a gratitude process. He works out regularly, and prepares for his workout with a few minutes of box breathing. After his workout, he does fifteen to twenty minutes of yoga, and then he does twenty-two minutes of focused breathing through his nose in a seated position.

He begins with a 3-6-6-3 pattern (inhale for a count of three; hold for a count of six; exhale for a count of six; hold for a count of three) for five minutes.

Then he slows it down to a 4-8-8-4 pattern for ten minutes (inhale four, hold eight, exhale eight, and hold four).

Then he moves to an even slower pattern of 5-10-10-5 for five minutes. And then he moves back to a pattern of 3-6-6-3 for two minutes. While breathing, Mark often engages in positive internal dialogue and visualizes success.

If you want to learn more about this great man, visit: http:// unbeatablemind.com/.

Master Tom Sotis: Elite Blade Fighter

Tom Sotis is the founder of AMOK! and one of the best blade fighters and self-defense instructors in the world. He works with some of the top government, military, and law enforcement agencies in the United States and worldwide.

This is a man who has been, as they say, "in the fire" many times, and so, he has knowledge and skills that can be learned and developed only by surviving life-and-death altercations a number of times.

Tom has the most remarkable powers of situational awareness, physical control, and subtle energy skills of almost anyone I have met. His system, AMOK!, has evolved continuously through constant experience, research, and development, and AMOK! is now the world's leading edged-weapons training company.

I met Tom many years ago through John Ebert, a mutual friend, breathing brother, and a fellow fire walker, along with Tony Robbins, who also teaches people to walk on hot coals, and I was immediately impressed with Tom's warrior spirit, his true grit, big heart, quick wit, sense of humor, and playfulness—such a refreshing and important balance to the extremely serious nature of his work.

Although Tom was cushioned by his mother's love, his father was extremely abusive. (This probably accounts for his early interest in the martial arts and his unusual calm, comfort, and grace in ultraviolent situations.)

When his son was born and Tom became a dad, he realized that he had some inner work to do in order not to pass on the negative patterns he'd inherited from his father. He didn't want to project his unresolved issues onto his son. That level of wisdom and caring made me an instant fan and a lifelong supporter.

It took only one breathing session for him to clean up years of emotional and psychological "stuff." And because of his level of skill, focus, and discipline, he was able to fine-tune his understanding of and approach to breathing, which resulted in a major breakthrough in his work as a blade fighter, along with a quantum leap in his teaching career.

I arranged for Tom to teach in the former Soviet Union in the early days of glasnost and perestroika. There he trained Russian special forces, presidential bodyguards, members of Spetsnaz, drug enforcement agents, hostage extraction teams, and private security personnel. To this day I meet people in Russia who remember his extraordinary demonstrations, and who share stories about their training with him.

You may not want to develop the extreme and specific abilities that guys like Tom have, but you can certainly make good use of the breathing exercises they teach and the principles that they apply.

Tom teaches a collection of breathing techniques that can be used with just about any physical sport or activity, from fencing to pocket billiards, from juggling to judo. I suggest that you pick one at a time, and practice it while engaged in your particular art, activity, routine, or workout.

Take in a full inhale and hold it in as long as you can.

Exhale fully and hold it out as long as you can.

Take a long, slow inhale until full.

Take a long, slow exhale until empty.

Break up your inhale into many tiny bits until full.

Break up your exhale into many tiny bits until empty.

Hyperventilate.

Try each of those breathing techniques in conjunction with a simple exercise or everyday activity to get a feel for them. For example, hyperventilate while you do the dishes, or break up your inhale and exhale into many small bits as you tie your shoes or get dressed. Work them into your training regimens (drills, routines, etc.) to challenge yourself and experience the benefits. If you would like to study directly with this master, visit: http://amok.global/.

Mikhail Ryabko: Russian Martial Arts Master

Mikhail Ryabko is a living legend in the world of Russian special forces. Very few people have seen the kind of action or survived the kinds of missions that he has, having led everything from antiterrorism raids to hostage-extraction teams. His unique approach to the fighting arts is based on breathing, relaxation, and believe it or not, love.

He and his leading teachers are true masters and are respected by the best martial artists in the world. I visited Master Ryabko at his training center in Moscow, and the longer I was with him, the more I wanted to hug him!

He called in his personal body worker, who gave me an hour-long massage session that frankly felt more like a torture session. If not for my stubborn ability to breathe and relax into pain, I doubt very much that I would have survived the experience. The more pain I felt, the more I turned to breathing and relaxation, and the more I relaxed, the more pain Ryabko's body worker inflicted on me. It was scary. My translator was unable to stay in the room, and our camera-person became ill just from watching. Later, I talked with Ryabko about pain, and he said: "Pain is fear. Period."

I have to agree about the connection between fear and pain. I couldn't tell the difference during my torture—I mean massage—session. When it was over, my entire body was buzzing with electricity for several hours. And I must admit, the next day I felt incredibly comfortable, fantastic in fact. And since then, my body has felt lighter, stronger, more relaxed, and more energized.

Ryabko also introduced me to his personal physician, who at over fifty years old is an extraordinary Ping-Pong player and is said to have one of the most powerful forehand shots in the world.

All of his top trainers demonstrate various unique and nearly superhuman abilities that seem unbelievable until you witness or experience them. The one thing they all share is their mastery of the Systema Breathing principles. Ryabko's partner, the Russian-born martial arts trainer Vladimir Vasiliev, explains systema breathing in his book *Let Every Breath* . . . Vasiliev immigrated to Canada and lives in Toronto. If you are a martial artist, he is someone you want to meet.

Like Ryabko, Vasiliev had an extraordinary military career. He is able to deliver the most amazing force with such ease and grace that he seems to defy the laws of physics and nature, when actually he is highly attuned to those laws and lives in harmony with them. He is a living example of a legendary master: possessed of uncanny and devastating fighting abilities and yet lighthearted, humble, and gentle, a truly loving and caring human being.

Here is my understanding and experience of the seven principles detailed in Vasiliev's book:

1. Practice nasal inhale and oral exhale: that means you breathe in through the nose and out through the mouth.

2. Lead with the breath and imagine a train. The breath should be like the engine: no part of your body—none of the cars—moves until the engine does.

3. Don't overbreathe and underbreathe. Develop the intuitive ability to allow the breath to perfectly meet and match your moment-to-moment energy and movement demands.

4. Master continuous breathing (this is the same breathing pattern that is used in Rebirthing Breathwork, discussed in Chapter 4).

5. Practice the perfect pendulum movement. This refers to the complete natural swing of the inhale and exhale cycles. It means not cutting either of them short, or forcing them beyond their natural length or speed.

6. Practice the principle of independence. Systema teaches that the breathing needs to be independent of any movements. And your strikes need to be equally powerful whether you are inhaling, exhaling, or holding your breath. This turns the old-school karate training of "exhaling when you strike" on its end.

7. Focus on complete relaxation. This is probably the subtlest yet most powerful Systema Breathing principle.

Here are some additional principles and practices, exercises and techniques that I have learned from Mikhail Ryabko:

Make use of breath sounds to focus: loud at first, softer over time, until ultimately inaudible.

Realize that breathing is not just mechanical or physiological; it does not begin and end with lungs.

Learn to infuse every cell—the whole body—with breath. Learn to breathe into and with every part of your body.

Always use relaxed breathing to transition from rest to activity, to avoid "cold starts." Learn to feel the pulse of your heartbeat everywhere in the body.

Play with tensing everything, starting from your feet all the way up to your face and head, while you inhale. Then release the tension from your head down to your feet during the exhale. Practice the reverse of this: tensing up on the exhale, relaxing on the inhale. Practice a complete cycle of inhale and exhale while tensing and relaxing.

Do breath-hold training at all points and phases of your exercises, moves, drills, and so on. Get comfortable with longer and longer holds. Learn to relax and tolerate air hunger.

Learn to pull yourself up with the breath: do sit-ups with straight spine and legs flat. Practice linking long inhales and long exhales to specific movements, series of movements, and various exercises and sets of exercises.

Learn to change your breathing pattern to overcome fatigue and endurance limits. Master the least amount of effort and tension during work and exercises.

Be creative about breath-body coordination. Practice inhaling into one part of the body and exhaling out of another. For example, breathe into one arm and breathe out the other; or breathe in through one leg and breathe out through the opposite arm.

Use "burst breathing" during long, strenuous exercises; for example during slow squats. Learn to "grab" pain or fatigue anywhere in the body through the nose and expel it through the mouth.

Learn to "bundle" the breaths. Do several squats or push-ups, for example, on a single in-breath or out-breath. Practice holding the breath at full, empty, and zero points during exercises.

Do partner breathing: focus on your own inner work while observing your partner. Copy or mirror each other's breathing. Practice breath walking. Synchronize breathing with your footsteps: 1-1, 2-2, 3-3, 4-4, etc.

If you sustain an injury or feel pain in a particular part of the body, breathe into and through that place to relieve the pain and to accelerate healing.

Boosting Your Creativity

Barnet Bain is a Hollywood producer, director, writer, filmmaker, and author of *The Book of Doing and Being*. As I read through his book, I couldn't help but notice how many times he mentioned breathing. He didn't give any specific instructions, but it was obvious that he was very aware of it, and that he used it consciously in his work. So I decided to meet him.

Since then, we have had some wonderful conversations about life, breathing, consciousness, and spirituality. During one of our conversations, Barnet pointed out that 98 percent of three-year-old children test as creative geniuses, yet only 2 percent of college graduates test as creative geniuses![11]

What happens to us? And how can we fix it? Barnet's answer: "When there's too much aliveness in the body, we evacuate the building. When feelings in the body become too strong, we abandon ship and take up residence in the head. Creativity is not born in the head; it comes as a gift from beyond. It's a heart thing. It's an emotional thing. It's a feeling thing. And so in the process of avoiding intense feelings, we cut ourselves off from the body, and therefore our creativity. The solution is to get back in touch with the body, to connect with feeling, and there is only one way to do that: breathing. Breathing is the whole deal!"

Brain science can help us to understand this. We have a reptilian brain that controls our fight-or-flight response. It also regulates other body systems, blood pressure, and so on. We have a limbic brain, a limbic system. This is responsible for emotional attunement, and attunement in general: play, fun, imagining, and so on. And we have the neocortex, the prefrontal cortex. It is in charge of the executive function, the logician.

Some people are born into unfortunate situations; for example, they have terrible parents. Even in the most fortunate situation, the fact is, no person can fully meet the needs of another human being. The problem begins something like this: you are an infant, days, weeks, or months old. Your mother is very loving, very attentive to you. Maybe you have a sibling, maybe she's on the phone, maybe she's busy with something else, and in that moment you crave attention. Where is she? She's gone! She's left me! This is not logical or rational, because your neocortex is not operational in that sense. It is a limbic response. It is preverbal. You experience an energetic abandonment. There is a severing of emotional attunement. The child feels it, and it is extremely painful.

So now you have this child who experiences a lack of attunement from his mother, his caregiver. Feelings of fear, abandonment, stress, and anxiety—an existential threat. It's too much. There's too much energy, there's too much aliveness—energetic aliveness—in that infant.

The feeling of abandonment is too much for that infant to handle. The system goes into overload. So what does the child do? The only thing it can do: it leaves the body, splits off, goes into a dissociative state. It leaves the body because there is too much body aliveness—distressing body aliveness.

We become more and more skillful at handling our abandonment as we grow up, and we train ourselves to check out, to leave. And there goes our creativity!

We begin with somatic aliveness. We begin with body awareness and limbic brain awareness, with them both operating. And we make a choice very early on to abandon ship. So now we look to restore our relationship to the primordial feminine energy that resides in the subconscious, which is the body. In order to reconnect with our creative energies, we must reconnect with the real feelings of aliveness in our body. The body holds everything. It never lies and it never forgets.

To regain our creativity, we need to relearn how to breathe. "But," as Barnet says, "now you might be a forty-two-year-old person living with a forty-two-year-old ghost!" So the challenge is that when you begin to breathe fully and freely, you reconnect with the same aliveness that terrified you once upon a time, that was too much for your little system to handle, and that caused you to escape.

What automatically happens is that when the breathing brings up these distressing feelings, your executive function takes over and you go into rational, logical thinking about medical facts and symptoms. You have a conceptual experience of your feelings instead of a real experience of them. Without the breath, you can only have a facsimile of feelings. For example, the "fear of loss" is not a feeling at all, it is a concept.

The mind tries to fit all experience into what it knows. Genuine innovation, real creativity, cannot happen in the head. It comes from the body, and you cannot get into the body without breathing. You'll just be moving the furniture around. Barnet pointed out that when Einstein was stuck on a problem, he got out of his head. He went sailing, or he played the violin, or he took a nap. In other words, he got into his body.

If you begin a breathing practice in a way that is simple and easy, then you will begin to gradually open up those original creative channels. You will begin to learn how to move the energy of aliveness through the body; you will start to see where there are blocks, places where the energy doesn't move, and you will become more intimate with your system.

Barnet reminds us that creativity is all about breathing. The problem is that your breathing "is like the pilot light on your oven: it's enough to keep you going, but not enough to cook anything."

"When you watch people hold their breath in the face of discomfort, you are seeing a map of the route they took to get out of town. When you live in your head instead of your body, it's like reading the lease on your apartment instead of living in it."

When you learn to get out of your head, energy that usually goes toward feeding the ego is available to heal the body and awaken creativity. When you learn to breathe, you release the residue of early life traumas, and this allows you to meet life's challenges with something other than the frightened three-year-old child in you.

❋ BREATHE NOW: CREATIVITY-BOOSTING PRACTICE

Here is the breathing practice that Barnet Bain teaches at his Creativity Camps and Creative Energy Trainings:

First, don't practice slow diaphragmatic breathing through your nose. "That's good for relaxation, for managing anxiety, and so on," Barnet says, "but it will not get you to a feeling of charged aliveness. It will not awaken your creative juices." He has people breathe through their mouth, into the upper chest and upper back.

He recommends that you start with five very big, fast full breaths. Put your hands over your collarbones and breathe into your upper chest. Breathe in and out through a wide-open mouth. Hold the breath in for a second or two, and then let it all out.

If you notice any uncomfortable sensations when doing this, then ground yourself by looking around and naming things: "white tablecloth," "computer on the desk," "plant on the shelf," "Dan in a black shirt," and so on.

Once you feel grounded, do another five or ten big, fast full breaths. Again breathe up under your collarbones, through your mouth. Pull in the breath, keep your mouth wide open, hold for a second or two, then let it all out through your mouth.

Gradually work up to fifty or sixty breaths like this, and you are well on your way to removing the biggest blocks to your creativity.

Everyday Breathing

One of the main points of breathwork is to integrate Breath Awareness and Conscious Breathing into our everyday lives. This adds a special quality to every experience. It keeps us connected to our spirit, it allows us to squeeze more juice out of life, and it helps us to be the best version of ourselves in all that we do.

Listening

During meetings or conversations, use your breath as a listening tool and to deepen your listening. Use your breath to take in a sense of the person's words. Also, notice what happens to your breathing when you are triggered by something that someone says, or when you are waiting to interject your own ideas in response. Feel your breath from your heart. Use the breath to listen from your heart.

Public Speaking

When it is your opportunity to speak, feel like you are using the breath to power your voice. Put yourself into a high-energy state and use your breath to channel this energy and to project your voice. Use the inhale to charge up, feel it fill you with confidence, and straighten and adjust your posture. Be conscious of breathing with your diaphragm, and feel your belly button moving toward your spine as you speak.

Boredom

If your mind starts to wander or you get bored, turn to your breath and use the opportunity to practice a mindfulness technique. Feel your feet on the floor. Feel the breath in your belly. Take in fresh energy and decide to focus. Become the watcher of your thoughts, judgments, and the nature of the mind wandering. Keep returning to the feeling of the breath in your belly.

Standing in Line

When you are in the middle of an unruly crowd, or you are waiting and there is nothing you can do about it, it's easy to get impatient and irritable. Instead, make a different choice. It's a wonderful opportunity to affect change in the world without anyone knowing. Focus on your heart, and expand your inhales as you breathe compassion toward yourself and toward the people around you, who are in the same predicament.

Busy Mind

Give yourself three long, slow expansive breaths, sending the breath low into your belly, filling it consciously. Focus on your body, on the physical feelings and sensations of expansion, as the breath overflows upward and fills your chest, then let the breath out slowly and very consciously. Then do a few minutes of paced breathing, five seconds in and five seconds out. End by practicing internal and situational awareness.

Yes!

When you breathe in, feel a "yes!" deep inside of you. Make the breath itself an expression of that "yes!" As you exhale say yes to giving; as you inhale say yes to receiving. Let every breath be a big yes to yourself, to your body, to life.

Breathing is the language of the soul. The way you breathe can express a yes or a no. Play with both. How do you breathe when you feel a no inside of you? How do you breathe when you feel a big yes? Notice the difference. Take some time right now to experience what a "yes" breath looks, feels, and sounds like.

4

BREATHING TO TRANSFORM YOUR SPIRIT

*In ancient times, there were the so-called spiritual men;
they mastered the universe, and controlled yin and yang.
They breathed the essence of life; they were independent
in preserving their spirit, and their muscles and flesh
remained unchanged. Therefore, they could enjoy a long
life, just as there is no end to heaven and earth.*

—*THE YELLOW EMPEROR'S CLASSIC OF INTERNAL MEDICINE*

anding at the airport in Delhi in August 1980 was a culture shock, and a shock in many other ways. The heat was practically unbearable, and we found ourselves having to step over hundreds of people camped out on the floor of the arrival hall. My wife, Louise, and my two boys, Danny and Dennis, were with me on our way to Babaji's ashram in Haidakhan. Meeting him was the most important part of becoming a Certified Rebirther in those days, because Leonard Orr believed that Babaji was the source and the inspiration for the rebirthing-breathwork movement. (Babaji is the legendary immortal yogi written about in *The Autobiography of a Yogi* by Paramahansa Yogananda, and meeting him in the flesh was the greatest blessing in my life.)[12]

My shock intensified when I asked one of the airport workers where the toilet was. Cheerfully pointing behind me, he answered—and in one sentence as if there was a logical connection—"Sorry, sir, no toilet; but we have a Space Invaders game!" Sure enough, there it was against the wall near the closed toilet.

As we made our way out to the street through the gauntlet of beggars and trinket sellers, and the barrage of rickshaw and taxi drivers vying for our business and tugging on our clothes and bags, I knew we were in for the adventure of our lives.

I decided to take a deep breath and settle into my new surroundings, but as the dust and smoke, the stench of human waste, and who knows what else, filled my nose and lungs, I decided that maybe it was better not to breathe too much in this city.

I learned how quickly I could adjust and adapt to uncomfortable things if I changed my focus, if I practiced acceptance. It really is amazing how comfortable we can become over time with almost anything, especially if we are not putting energy into resisting or complaining, as long as we are willing to surrender to what is—as it is. And that's exactly what I was doing: practicing acceptance, using the experience and the situation to strengthen my spiritual muscles.

I woke up the next morning, feeling quite at home in those strange surroundings. I went out to the garden and was greeted by my friend and teacher Leonard Orr. He asked me how I was doing, and I said "Great!" I really was feeling very good, unusually good, and for no apparent reason at all.

"What are we doing today?" I asked.

"Let's go meet Indira Gandhi!"

Thinking it was a joke, I played along: "Sure. Let's go knock on the door of the White House!"

"No, I'm serious," he said. "Let's go."

India, we were told, was a magical place, and I had already decided to surrender and go with the flow, so the two of us set out to find a taxi. Leonard told our driver that we wanted to meet the prime minister. "So you want to go to the prime minister's office, then?" the taxi driver asked. I said "Yes, that's right!" just to confirm that I was in on this crazy idea too.

We ended up at a big government building, and then at a receptionist's desk, talking to a clerk. He listened to our request and smiled politely as he wrote down our names. After a few minutes, he said thank you and told us to: "Please come back tomorrow at 8 A.M."

We arrived at exactly eight the next day and found a line of several hundred people stretching from the building entrance, down the street, and around the corner. I remember thinking: *maybe she comes out every day and waves to people*. We made our way to the end of the line and waited. After about thirty minutes, as the line kept growing longer and wider, I noticed an Indian man with a clipboard making his way along the row of people, shouting something. As he came closer, I realized that he was calling our names: "Dan Brulé? Leonard Orr?"

Leonard raised his hand like he was taking an oath and I waved the guy over to us. He took us to the front of the line, in through the door, and to the same reception desk as the day before. Leading us to a room with a large conference table, he said: "Please wait here."

Leonard and I sat in silence. My six-year-old son Dennis sat on my lap, his legs dangling as he quietly played with my shirt collar. Two women from our group had also joined us on the adventure, and they were quietly whispering to each other. I heard Leonard take a soft, conscious breath, which reminded me to do the same. And in walked Indira Gandhi!

"Good morning. Thank you so much for coming," Mrs. Gandhi said. Would you like some water, or some tea?" At first, I was speechless; we were being greeted and waited on by the prime minister of India!

She had such a warm demeanor and a genuine smile. Her skin glowed, and she was so relaxed and gracious. And her sari was perfectly white and without a single wrinkle.

I started the conversation by saying: "This is so amazing! I have been trying to meet the president of the United States my whole life without success, and yet after only two days in the country, I am sitting with you."

"India is a magical place," she said.

She had come into the room carrying a stack of documents, signing them as we talked. We sat with her for more than forty-five minutes that day, discussing yoga and the schools in India, how they compared to the schools in America. As we sat there, I became obsessed with and focused on one thing: her breathing. There was something fascinating about it—it was so subtle, yet so alive. It felt like I was looking at breathing for the first time.

I knew that our breathing expresses and reflects our changing thoughts and feelings, but I had never realized just how much it did so, or with such detail. As she made her way through the stack of documents, signing some, scribbling notes on others, I watched her fingers on the pen; I could feel it in her hand. I could feel the movement of her breath under her collarbones and the sensations of it.

I began to mirror every breath she took, and as I did, I could feel what was happening within her. I was experiencing her thoughts and her emotions. I had such a powerful sense of certainty that I was experiencing a clear and unmistakable connection to the inner world of another being in a way I had never experienced before.

Mrs. Gandhi's breathing would change and move with each document she reviewed or studied. Sometimes her breath shot high in her chest in a dramatic way, and other times it was so subtle and light as to be barely perceptible. A few times it dropped deep into her lower belly with such force and power I thought she was about to get up; other times it settled there as if lightly coming home to rest.

Sometimes her breath would speed up, and sometimes it would slow down—sometimes suddenly, sometimes gradually. And sometimes she seemed to enter an endless pause as she studied some details or thought through an idea. I could tell when her attention moved on, because her breath did so in the same moment.

Riding her breath from this conscious state, I could tell which documents were mere bureaucratic formalities that simply required her signature, and which ones moved her in a deeper way. For some, there was clearly no emotional investment, no thought of liking or not liking, and no change in her breathing. But then as she reviewed another one, her breath would pause, as if she was having second thoughts, thinking through her decision. Another time I got the clear feeling that she was conceding to something or someone in order to resolve an issue, an uncomfortable but necessary trade-off. Meanwhile she showed no changes on her face, in her posture, in the tone of her voice, or in our conversation. Only her breathing gave her away.

For the first time, I really understood the value of Breath Awareness, knowing it with certainty on a cellular level. Maybe there was something special about her, or maybe I was more open somehow. In any case, in her presence I was able to access a deep sense of intuition, and since then, I have viewed breathing in a very different way. We all have remarkable inborn abilities waiting to be discovered or uncovered. Breathing is the key to bringing them alive in us.

And so, now, let's go deeper into the practice so you can experience some of these higher abilities for yourself.

Deepening Your Practice of Breath Awareness

In order to master the art and science of breathwork, you will need to develop a very conscious relationship with your breath by delving deeper into the practice of Breath Awareness, which I also call breath watching. This practice is the first and most important element in breathwork, the key and the first step toward breath mastery.

Most of the time you are not conscious of your breathing. It's happening outside of your awareness. To compensate for this, reclaim greater awareness, and regain balance and stillness, begin to meditate on your breathing. We can practice Breath Awareness anytime, anywhere, for a moment or two, or for an hour or more. The more conscious we become of our breath, the more conscious we become of everything: our thoughts and feelings, our habits and patterns, our posture, our behavior, other people's energy, our surroundings, and so on. The more Breath Awareness you have, the more benefits you will get from the breathing exercises or techniques in this book.

Commit to putting aside some time for breath watching. Ten minutes is good. Twenty minutes is better. See that you won't be disturbed or interrupted. Be sure to leave some time for yourself afterward, to move and stretch, write in your journal, enjoy a cup of tea, or do something else that you love. Do not underestimate the value of this simple practice. It has profound benefits, both immediate and long term.

✽ BREATHE NOW: BREATH AWARENESS PRACTICE

The main thing about the practice of Breath Awareness is that you are not doing the breathing. You are not breathing in any particular way. You are allowing the breath to come and go by itself, the way it wants. You are letting the body breathe itself. You're just an impartial observer, a detached witness. You are watching and feeling the breath breathe you.

If the breath moves through your nose, focus your attention on the feelings and sensations at the tip of your nose as the air passes in and out. If you are breathing through your mouth, notice the feelings and sensations of the air as it passes over your lips and tongue, cooling the roof of your mouth and swirling in your throat.

You can also focus on the feelings and sensations in your chest or belly as the breath moves in and out. In other words, you can track the breathing moment to moment by being aware of what the breath touches and what moves in your body when you breathe.

When your mind wanders, and it will; when you get caught up in thinking, and you will; or when something else pulls your attention away, simply and gently come back to your breathing: focus totally on your next breath. Don't get angry or frustrated with yourself or your restless monkey mind; simply return to watching the breath.

After the exercise, review your experience. What feelings, sensations, or movements did you notice? Where? How would you describe or characterize your breathing pattern: slow, quick, deep, shallow, smooth, chaotic, forced, natural, effortless?

If breathing is the language of the soul, if your breathing reflects and expresses your relationship to life, what does your breathing pattern tell you about yourself, the state of your being, and your attitude toward life?

Do this practice daily, as part of your morning ritual. And take it into your daily activities. Stop from time to time during the day and simply observe your breathing.

How do you breathe when—

someone is insulting you?
someone is praising you?

a problem has you going around and around in your head?

you are conscious of your heart space?

you are angry, afraid, or upset?

you feel peaceful, loving, and kind?

you are putting a key in a door?

you are trying to remember something?

you are late and stuck in traffic?

you are trying to solve a math problem?

you are enjoying music?

you are in pain?

you are having an orgasm?

you are approaching a serious encounter or an important event?

you are dealing with intense emotions or a stressful experience?

nothing is going your way?

you are in the flow, when you are in the zone?

Begin to pay attention, not only to your own breathing but also to the breathing in others: people you meet in public and in private, those with whom you work and play. Pay attention to their breath when they speak, move, complain, celebrate, watch TV, listen to music. Notice their breathing when they are angry, nervous, embarrassed. We often learn a lot about ourselves by observing others.

Spiritual Breathing

The breath is often overlooked and underestimated in our search for the source and meaning of life. Yet the Bible tells us clearly: "And the Lord God formed man of the dust of the earth, and breathed into his nostrils the breath of life; and man became a living soul" (Genesis 2:7).

I don't want to get too religious on you here, but you can deepen your connection to the source of life in you, or even find your way back to God if you have become lost, by turning to the breath . . . You can awaken to what is referred to in Hebrew as *neshemet ruach chayim*: "the spirit of life within the breath." The fact is there is something more to the air that we breathe than just the air. It is the life-giving principle that is both contained within and can be expressed through the breath. Many languages use the same word for air, wind, or breath as they do for life, vital energy, spirit, or the animating principle of life: chi, ki, prana, and energy. This inner breath runs through body, mind, and soul.

A Course in Miracles, by the Foundation for Inner Peace, a book about spiritual transformation, teaches us that: "A universal theology is impossible, but a universal experience is not only possible, it is necessary." I believe that this universal experience is the breath, is breathing.[13]

Spiritual breathing is to psychosomatic illness what penicillin is to infection. Spiritual breathing is the quickest way to clear your head, settle your stomach, calm your nerves, and open your heart. It will uplift you, center you, and ground you in your being. Spiritual breathing opens your heart to love and fills your body with light and life.

The breath is the fire of the heart—the heart of love. The Quakers have a wonderful tradition. At their Sunday service, people simply sit in silence and meditation, waiting, open to inspiration. And when it comes, when the spirit moves them, they speak. They say their piece (peace). They also believe that now and then we need to open all the doors and windows of our heart and soul, and let the spirit of God blow through us.

Breathwork is a spiritual technology of awakening. When you work with the breath, you automatically develop a sense of spirituality and spiritual abilities. On the physical, material level we have solids, liquids, and gases. To play with breath is to play with the subtlest form of matter. That's why people who have mastered spiritual breathing can accomplish so much on the level of subtle energies. Spiritual breathing makes it clear that the original creative life force energy that built our bodies in the womb is still available to us, to maintain and even rebuild the body.

Yoga is the science of union (with God). And yoga holds as a central truth that breath is the connection, the bridge, between mind and body, between the visible and the invisible. Breath connects us to each other, and it connects all of us to God, nature, and existence.

Each of us must walk our own unique path. And that is the empowering aspect of breathwork: no one can do it for you! Every breath we take can be a prayer, an invitation, and a genuine demonstration of our faith. Every breath can be an active expression of trust, or forgiveness, or gratitude.

We are all breathing the same breath. The breath that is in me now was in someone else earlier, and it will be in the bird flying overhead tomorrow. It was in the dog walking down the street yesterday. This is not just a pretty philosophy; it is a fact. We literally share the same breath with everyone who has ever lived and breathed on this earth. Some of the same atoms and molecules of air that were breathed by Jesus, Moses, and Buddha are flowing through you and me right now.

If you really want to touch the deepest realities of life, and to reach the highest states of consciousness, then you will have to awaken to the breath. It is the path, the doorway, and the connection to your essence, your core, and your soul.

I like to think that there is an angel of breath at work on the planet. This angel brings fire and light to everyone on the spiritual path. Evolutionary contractions in the form or natural disasters, social upheaval, wars, and rumors of wars are doing the work of pushing spiritual seekers out of their comfort zone and into the dynamic working zone of spiritual awakening, purification, and rebirth.

I believe everyone is born a spiritual master. But we forget, we lose touch with our essence, our purpose, and our source. You can begin to incorporate the life of spirit back into your body and mind simply by breathing in a conscious way. Practice breathing in ways that are peaceful, accepting, trusting, loving, grateful, forgiving, inviting, and surrendering. Incorporating these attributes with spiritual breathing makes manifesting them in reality easy and effortless.

More than knowing, believing, or doing it, when you are breathing it, you are *living* it. You are *being* it. Opening and relaxing the breath is like opening the doors to your soul. Use your breath to allow every fiber of your being to be bathed in the life force that flows from the source. Spiritual breathing has been called a biological experience of divine energy, a cellular experience of God.

It takes courage to live a unique and inspired life. It requires that you turn to your own inner truth, which is reflected and expressed with every breath you take. Breathing is like a language: "the language of the soul." And you need to begin to communicate with your soul in the only language that it knows: the language of the heart and love.

It takes courage to follow your heart and walk your own path. There is such a powerful illusion of security in following the crowd, or in following the way of the great ones. But if you are walking someone else's path, you are walking the wrong path. It doesn't matter how great the one was who created the path, or how many millions of people believe it is the right one. At some point you will need to walk alone. Your only companion, your only guide, will be your own breath.

Spiritual breathing can take you to the eye of the storm in your life. Spiritual breathing can help you to balance yin and yang, peace and power, rhythm and harmony. You can learn about yourself from the breath itself. Through Conscious Breathing, you can learn to follow your bliss!

The ultimate benefits of spiritual breathing may seem inconceivable to many people. For example, Leonard Orr, the father of Rebirthing Breathwork, believes that it actually offers us a path to physical immortality, to biological immortality. Conscious Breathing, he says, is a way that we can begin to include the physical body into the eternal life of the spirit. I have a hunch that he's on to something. Leonard has written many books over the years. They are all in my library. One of the most fascinating is *Breaking the Death Habit*.[14]

Whatever your aspirations are, however lofty or mundane, theoretical or practical, you can't miss by turning to the breath. You can't go wrong by inviting God, or your own spirit, or life itself, to take part in your mission. Feel the sensations of breath, the movement of life in you. Be a witness. Pay attention to what is happening inside of you in each moment.

Add to that the willingness to let go, to surrender. And then begin to conspire with the life force that surrounds and permeates everything in existence. Breathe this life force consciously. Feel the expansion and contraction of that life. Celebrate the presence and flow of that life in you, as you. Marvel at the miracle of life and open to the mystery of life that can be revealed to you with each breath.

Seek out others who are committed to breath mastery. Share your experience. We all have to walk our own path, but we can walk together with others for a time. My burning belief is that no one is free until we are all free. And whenever any one of us becomes totally free, we make it that much easier for everyone else to become liberated! We are all connected, so we help ourselves best when we serve others, and we help others most when we serve ourselves.

Consciously breathe peace and love, freedom and safety, energy and aliveness, love and light. Watch the world within you and the world around you change forever!

Spiritual breathing is the name of my favorite practice, my idea of the highest application of breathwork. It's based on the fact that whenever energy and consciousness come together, something is created. That is the creative process: bringing together energy and consciousness. Spiritual breathing means joining the breath with every creative and functional aspect of ourselves—using everything at our disposal. It's about being total.

"One pointedness" is an important principle I first learned from aikido, a Japanese martial art. It means bringing mind and body together. When we do that, a powerful force emerges. That's how martial artists break bricks, and how skinny little old guys can throw big strong young guys around the room with ease.

With spiritual breathing, we bring together body, mind, and breath, and as a result, an even greater force emerges: a healing, creative force for transformation and evolution.

Everything begins in consciousness. The computer I am using right now began as an idea in someone's head. Look around. Almost everything that you can see or touch in the physical world first took form in someone's consciousness, and from there, with faith and passion, determination and action, it found its way out into physical reality and into your world.

Some people would say that the entire physical universe, and that nature itself, along with you and me and everything that exists, began as a thought, a desire, an idea, in the mind of God.

The more passion, enthusiasm, and focused energy and awareness we bring to whatever we imagine or desire or intend to do, the more likely we will create it, attract it, or do it.

Spiritual breathing is about focusing on a high spiritual principle, and then pouring as much passion as we can into it with every breath.

In spiritual breathing, the goal is to make each breath as thick and juicy as we can, as wholesome and delicious and delightful as possible. It means bringing every level of our being into the moment-to-moment practice and process of Conscious Breathing.

There are five levels of being or forms of expression that we can bring consciously to each breath: thoughts, images, sounds, movement, and emotions. They are ways you can be creative with your breathwork practice. Play with them now.

1. Thoughts: These can include words, phrases, affirmations, statements, mantras, prayers. Mentally repeat a high-frequency word or phrase with each breath. For example: "love," "I am loved, I am loving"; "peace," "I am peaceful"; "joy," "I radiate joy"; "health," "I am healthy"; "freedom," "I am always already free." Choose any beautiful word or phrase, and breathe the energy and feeling of it into every cell of your body.

2. Images: Create pictures in your mind, visual representations of the words or phrases you are focusing on. Imagine the face of your beloved or a beautiful scene, or imagine a bright light or a beautiful color that fits the word or phrase that you have chosen. Images of loved ones, family, friends, teachers, and students; their smiles, their words, their energy come to me when I focus on love and peace and joy.

3. Sounds: Children love to make sounds when they are playing or imagining something. Use breath sounds (*oooh . . . ahhhh . . . eeeehh . . . ohhh . . . mmmm . . . ssshhh . . . aum . . . vrroom*). Make any enjoyable sound that resonates with the image or thought that you are playing with while you breathe. Breath sounds . . . wind noises . . . ocean noises . . .

4. Movement: Move your body in some pleasurable way. Use your body to express and reflect what you are feeling and imagining while you breathe. Do something with your fingers, hands, and arms; your head, neck, eyes, spine, toes. Let the breath move your body, and let your body move the breath.

5. Emotions: In the same way that you can generate a thought, an image, a sound, or a movement, you can generate an emotion. Put feeling into the process. Gratitude is a very powerful emotion, and we don't even need a reason to generate it. Be dramatic in your expression. Send a clear message to your subconscious. Leave no doubt to anyone who may be watching that you are enjoying something amazing!

In what other ways can you bring the totality of your being into each breath? Begin breathing, and then strive to bring in as much of your body, mind, heart, and soul as you can to the process. Infuse each breath with the highest, most beautiful, powerful thoughts, images, sounds, movements, and emotions you can conjure up. Be total and spontaneous. Be creative. Be passionate. Open yourself to ecstasy!

❋ BREATHE NOW: SPIRITUAL BREATHING PRACTICE

The power of spiritual breathing lies in its simplicity: just add a little stretch to your inhale. Consciously expand your in-breath a bit more than usual. Gently take in a deeper, fuller breath than normal. And then deliberately let go into a long, soothing sigh of relief.

As you exhale, feel yourself or imagine yourself dropping down into your center—as if you are leaving the surface and settling into a deeper part of yourself. Leave behind what you think, how you feel, what you do. Let go of the mundane world, your daily activities, your habits and patterns, your routines. Just for a moment, let go of your thoughts about right and wrong, should and shouldn't, must and must not . . .

Drop down to a place before and beyond your conditioning. Let go of your history, the past . . . And at the same time, feel your borders softening . . . Imagine the boundaries of your body dissolving . . . Imagine or feel yourself radiating light from your heart, like the sun . . . expanding outward . . . merging with everything and everyone . . . Dropping down, to settle into your center, while also expanding and radiating outward to merge with everything and everyone.

We are bigger than we think. We are greater than we have been led to believe. As you breathe, give yourself permission to sense that you are an infinite eternal being. The cosmos is within us as well as around us. We are all connected. There is only one life, one energy, one being in the universe—one being, being you and me. We can use the breath to experience the state of nonduality, to escape the illusion of separation.

It might be important to note here that language is extremely important and useful, but it can also be quite limiting, and it can even put us in a mental trap. Some things are difficult, if not impossible, to put into words. That's why in breathwork we focus on feelings, we focus on the heart.

Every cell in your body thinks that it is an individual separate entity unto itself, and it is: it moves by itself, takes in food and excretes waste, communicates with other cells, and yet it is part of an organ. And that organ thinks it is a separate individual thing, and it is: your heart is not your kidney, your kidney is not your liver. And yet these organs are part of a system, and that system thinks it is unique and individual and separate, and yet that system is part of a larger one . . . And on and on it goes forever.

On the other hand, if you look into a single cell, you will find smaller particles. Crack those open, and you find even smaller ones, and on and on it goes forever. You are part of an endless eternal infinite reality. You are that reality.

✺ BREATHE NOW: MERGING WITH EXISTENCE

Imagine that when you inhale, the breath travels to you from somewhere beyond the universe, it flows to you from across time and space. It flows through you, and when you exhale it continues on its eternal cosmic journey. When you breathe in, imagine that the breath also arises from within you, from the center of every cell in your body. Let your borders dissolve. Let your ego dissolve. Don't try to wrap your mind around this practice. Get into your heart. Be like a child, be imaginative, be creative. Merge with existence.

Welcome to spiritual breathing!

Introduction to Rebirthing Breathwork

I've mentioned my friend Leonard Orr, the creator and founder of the worldwide Rebirthing Breathwork movement. He has spent over forty years of his life spreading the healing power of this technique, which is also known as "connected breathing."

Rebirthing is a direct road to spiritual breakthroughs, opening you up to an extraordinarily liberating energy experience. And because I have experienced so many amazing results with this technique, I really have to share a bit more, an offering to whet your curiosity and hopefully encourage you to explore it on your own. Since practicing this technique for even a few minutes can trigger a powerful healing or transformational process, sometimes it's best to have a coach, facilitator, or at least a breathing buddy nearby when you experiment.

The Rebirthing Breathwork technique is as simple as it is powerful. Here are the basics: the inhale is active and the exhale is passive. Pull the inhale in consciously and let the exhale go quickly and completely (the key phrase here is "let go").

There are no pauses or gaps between the inhale and the exhale, between the exhale and the inhale. No holding, no hesitating. The breaths are connected in a smooth, steady rhythm.

Once you begin, breathe continuously: inhale merging with the exhale, exhale blending seamlessly into the next inhale. The breath is turning like a wheel. Just keep breathing and relaxing into and through whatever you feel, whatever comes up.

From time to time, you can take a long, expansive inhale and give yourself a big, exaggerated sigh of relief, then go right back into the connected rhythm.

Use the same channel to breathe through. That is, breathe either in and out the nose or in and out the mouth, but do not breathe in the nose and out the mouth.

To learn more about Rebirthing Breathwork, check out Leonard's website: www.leonardorr.com.

Breathing with Ram Dass

Ram Dass is the author of *Be Here Now, Journey of Awakening, Grist for the Mill,* among others. Over the years, through his life and his work, and because of him, millions of Americans have discovered Eastern philosophy and spirituality, yoga and meditation. I'm happy and grateful to say that I am one of them.

One day while in X-ray school, I overheard a conversation in the cafeteria at Boston City Hospital about a Harvard professor who had gone to India and found a guru. When he came back, he walked around the Harvard University campus wearing an Indian robe, with mala beads around his neck, chanting mantras.

Talk about far out! His name was Dr. Richard Alpert, but he was now known as Ram Dass (He said his father jokingly referred to him as Rum Dum!). Ram Dass would be giving a talk that night in Cambridge, and I decided on the spot that I had to meet him.

After work, still dressed in my hospital greens, I found myself in the basement of the Harvard Bookstore, which had a New Age hippie, churchlike atmosphere. The room was packed. In order to get in, I had to disturb the last three rows of devotees who were piously sitting in meditation. Once I was able to squeeze in and close the door behind me, I realized that I was the only one standing, the only one not sitting in the lotus position, the only one not looking appropriately spiritual. The smell of incense filled the air. I felt so weird and out of place. I felt trapped.

Ram Dass had stopped talking when I distracted everyone with my noisy entrance. After a few moments, he resumed speaking softly and slowly, and his talk . . . was filled . . . with . . . pregnant . . . pauses. Catching his words and letting the meaning sink in was like impatiently waiting for filtered coffee to be ready: drip . . . drip . . . drip . . . I like instant coffee, from a drive-through window! My mind was racing, and at the same time I was bored to death with all this silly divine love "woo-woo" and guru nirvana enlightenment stuff!

Yet he felt very sincere to me so I was trying to catch what he was saying, but all I could hear was my own mental chatter—my mind reacting to everything he said. I was restless, fidgeting constantly, shifting from one foot to the other. I wanted a cigarette! I began to hope that someone would try to push open the door behind me so I could let them in and make my escape. I was torturing myself.

To make things worse, Ram Dass kept interrupting his talk to eat grapes. And he couldn't just eat the damn grapes. No! He had to pick up each one very slowly, and he had to deliberately turn it in his fingers and look at it ever so lovingly. He had to bring it slowly to his lips and chew it ever so carefully; and then with his eyes closed, swallow it, blissfully feeling it slowly slide down his throat.

I was getting to the point where I simply couldn't bear it. Disturb everyone or not, I had to get the hell out of there! My mind supported and encouraged me: "Yes, let's go home," it said. "You'll never see any of these people again anyway, so who cares if you disturb them?" In that very moment, Ram Dass looked directly at me. I felt like a deer caught in his headlights! He began to speak directly to me, or so it seemed. It was over forty-five years ago, and yet it feels like yesterday. I remember every word he said:

"You were born at this time, in this place, in this family, in this socioeconomic setting . . ."

Then he reached for a grape! My breathing stopped as he took forever to eat that freakin' grape! And it only started again when he finished his sentence:

". . . for a purpose."

Then he went on to say what he later wrote in his book: "And everything you do, everything that happens to you, is grist for the mill of realizing that purpose."

Then he said, "Let's do this: when you breathe in, think to yourself, 'The power of God is within me,' and when you breathe out, think to yourself, 'The grace of God surrounds me.' Breathing in: 'the power of God is within me,' and breathing out: 'the grace of God surrounds me.'"

Driving home that night on the Southeast Expressway, it wouldn't stop, and I couldn't shut it off. It was impossible to breathe without remembering those words, and impossible to remember those words without breathing. I was suddenly back in the first-grade classroom, and God was breathing into me. Those words reawakened in me the glorious feelings from that day with the pastor. Thank you, Rum Dum! I will always love you, and I will always be grateful.

✳ BREATHE NOW: UNITING THOUGHT AND INTENTION

Take the time to focus on what is most important to you. Focus on what gives you the most wonderful feeling. Put that into a word or a phrase or a sentence and begin to breathe it into every cell of your body.

Be creative! Breathe your intention. Take five minutes right now to do this exercise. Use the phrases that Ram Dass suggested. Or create or choose your own empowering statement, affirmation, declaration, wish, or prayer. Choose your own soothing or strengthening words.

Make sure the words you choose lift you up or calm you down. Make sure they inspire or motivate you to be your best; bring you peace; are wonderful thoughts and beautiful feelings. Make sure you are creating or inviting a reality that you can live with forever; that you are breathing as you do this thinking process. And make sure you let yourself feel the feelings that these words bring up in you.

What are the most beautiful words you could speak to yourself? What are the most beautiful words you could speak to someone else? What do you wish for yourself and for the world? What are your highest aspirations? What is your heart's grandest desire? What is your purpose, your mission in life? What is your fondest dream? A heartfelt intention fueled by the power of the breath can change everything.

This is a creative process. You are bringing together consciousness and energy, thought and action: this is the essence of creativity. Be careful what you think about while you breathe, because every breath you take gives life force energy to what you hold in consciousness. As they say: "thought is creative," and "thoughts become things."

Vipassana and Insight Meditation

Ram Dass originally turned me on to Buddhist meditation, and Milton Young, my mentor at UMass Dartmouth, inspired me to dive deep into the practice, convincing me to do a number of intensive vipassana meditation retreats. It was just what I needed as I tried to get my footing after leaving the military. And I was fortunate to live within driving distance of the Insight Meditation Center in Barre, Massachusetts.

I studied with Jack Kornfield, Joseph Goldstein, and Sharon Salzberg, and that led me to meeting the venerable Ajahn Chah. Looking back now, I realize what a rare opportunity, what a blessing it was to study and practice with such a great master and to be guided by such powerful, sincere, and genuine spiritual teachers so early in my learning process.

Vipassana meditation is a simple technique where you sit quietly and watch your breath. While sitting for hours on end paying attention to your breath gives you sore knees and a sore butt, it can also result in powerful spiritual breakthroughs. The practice is like training a wild monkey. You put a collar on it, give it a short leash, and tie it to a post. It kicks and screams and tries everything to break free and run wild. But after some time it, it gives up, lets go, and learns to sit still. Then you don't even need the post and leash anymore. Vipassana is monkey mind training. I am so grateful to my teachers, and to myself, for practicing it long enough to come out of the dark tangled jungle of my head and into the bright inner sky of my heart.

I cannot recommend vipassana meditation enough. Deciding to practice it was one of the wisest decisions I ever made. It still helps me at every step on my path of breath mastery. As with any spiritual practice involving a lineage, it's a good idea to get as close to the source of it as possible. So, I suggest you do a Google search, consult with your intuition, and choose a teacher with a long history of practice in this method, and then dive into it fully. You will be glad you did.

Here's the practice: sit comfortably but erect in a chair or on a cushion. Turn your attention to the breath, to the feelings and sensations of the air coming in and going out. Nothing to do: just observing, just being consciously aware of your breathing. When your mind wanders—and it will—just return your attention to the breathing. Simple. Do this mindfulness practice for ten or twenty minutes right now, and make it a regular practice.

Awaken Your Intuition

Some people talk about intuition as a feeling, or sometimes an inner voice. Many people wonder how to differentiate between our intuitive voice and the voice in our head, the difference between our heart and our mind, between natural wisdom and rational mental chatter. Fortunately, that is one of the most beautiful benefits of breathwork: it gives us a way to know and feel the difference.

Imagine a horse and rider. To become an expert rider, you have to learn to work with the horse, learn its personality and build trust. When we come into harmony with the horse, our ride is smooth and graceful. When we fight it or are out of sync, the ride hurts, it's tiring, and it is a mutual struggle. You are either in the flow with the horse or not. When a rider and a horse are in tune, when they flow together, it's an exhilarating experience, and it's beautiful and even thrilling to behold.

When you learn to ride the breath, when you can flow with it, when you are in tune with it, you have established a real and practical connection to your intuition. There's no confusion, and there's no faking it: your ride is smooth and in sync. You have a clear sense of having effortlessly harnessed a tremendous power. You respond to that power, and that power responds to you. The rider can sense what the horse needs, and the horse responds to the rider's subtlest wishes. The relationship is beautiful; it's awesome.

When we breathe in, air comes from the outside into our lungs, but something else happens: energy seems to rise up from within us and it fills us. It feels like the surge of an ocean. We have a sense of relaxing and opening and giving space to this energy.

When this happens, we are coming into harmony with our intuition, and it feels as if the breath is breathing us! When we develop this kind of relationship with the breath, we find ourselves in the right place at the right time, doing and saying the right things in the right way.

Intuition is a sense of being in the zone, or in the flow, in a state of oneness, of clarity and simple ease. The best athletes and artists, the greatest musicians and soldiers know this state very well. They may or may not be conscious of it at the time, but when they are performing at their peak, energy is rising up from within them, flowing through them from beyond, and it is being effortlessly directed perfectly from within, with ease and grace.

✹ BREATHE NOW: THE DANCE OF BREATH

When you are breathing intuitively, it feels like a dance. You and the breath are one. Yes, there is a leader and a follower, but when the partners are in the flow, that distinction seems to disappear.

As you breathe in, feel the breath wanting to open, stretch, and expand you. Move with the breath. Deliberately relax and open and give it space. You are being a good dance partner.

Now notice that when you open and relax yourself during the inhale, the breath, like a good dance partner, pours into you and fills the spaces that you create. Notice that just creating a bit of space between your teeth allows air to pour in more easily and more freely. Pull the air into yourself with the inhale, but also imagine pulling it, or letting it rise up from within you at the same time. Let these two movements or air and energy meet in your heart—the seat of your intuition. And on the exhale relax and let go completely. Drop down into your center and expand and radiate out beyond your borders at the same time.

Maintain as much of that open relaxation as you can as you take in the next breath. Feel yourself opening and expanding and giving space to the breath and energy. Feel yourself letting go and dropping down, surrendering to the flow. As you breathe, play with speed, volume, rate, and intensity. And remember to keep relaxing and letting go. Are you breathing the breath, or is the breath breathing you? Get lost in that dance!

Spiritual Energy in Breathwork

When people talk about energy, I often wonder what they are really talking about. We know about prana, chi, ki, life force, and spirit. This is the energy in the breath that we are learning to feel, tap, move, and direct with our breath. Is this what they are talking about? When people say they feel energy, that they are sensitive to energy, what do they really mean? Here is my understanding:

When a boat moves through water, it makes waves. When you feel those waves, are you feeling the boat? When energy moves through the body and mind, it makes waves: feelings and sensations, thoughts, and images. When you experience these things, are you experiencing the energy? No, you are experiencing the waves the energy makes when it passes through you. You are experiencing the reactions of your mind-body system to the energy.

When people tell me that they are very sensitive, I often wonder, are they really sensitive, or are they simply hyperreactive? It seems to me that as long as your body and mind are reacting, you cannot really be sensitive. It is not until the body and mind stop reacting that we are able to experience the energy directly. Not until we stop reacting can we be truly sensitive.

That's why in breathwork we practice three fundamental spiritual principles:

1. Nonjudgment
2. Nonresistance
3. Nonattachment

Sound familiar? These principles were taught by the Buddha and by many other awakened ones. They represent a spiritual antidote to the causes of suffering. I spent many years practicing nonjudgment, nonresistance, and nonattachment. It is still an ongoing practice.

Then one day I realized that all three of these things were reactions. **Judging is a reaction, resistance is a reaction, and attachment is a reaction.** So here is a shortcut: practice nonreaction. I have distilled my practice down to nonreaction. This is one of the secrets of breath mastery as well as self-mastery, and it may be the key to self-realization and ultimate liberation.

There is a beautiful analogy related to consciousness during breathwork, and that is the analogy of water. We could ask: "What would Jesus do?" Or "What would love do?" Or we could ask: "What would water do?" When you throw a stone in a river or a pond, the water reacts perfectly. It doesn't overreact, and it doesn't underreact. Our goal is to have that kind of mind and that kind of body.

Moreover, water has two very interesting properties: it is transparent and it is reflective. I can see through the water to the bottom; I can see the fish midway down. I can also see myself reflected on the surface of the water. That is, if the water is pure and still, calm and unmoving. This is the kind of consciousness that we need to develop. And breathwork gives us a way of doing exactly that: developing that high, refined, expanded, and sublime quality of consciousness.

As you have noticed, I use the terms "awareness" and "consciousness" very often and interchangeably, as if they are synonymous. I'm sure some would argue that they are not, and they may be correct, but to a great extent, for our purposes, they are the same.

I heard a story many years ago about two of my favorite teachers: the Buddha and Patanjali. We already know quite a bit about the Buddha. Patanjali may not be as well known. He is considered to be the father of yoga. He did not invent yoga, but he took all the yogic wisdom of his day and organized it into a system called the *Yoga Sutras*. Patanjali and the Buddha never met. They came from different cultures and different times, but they were clearly spiritual cousins, even brothers.

Both the Buddha and Patanjali had the same mission in life: to find the cause and the cure of suffering. And if you look at the list of the causes of suffering that the Buddha identified, and compare it to the list that Patanjali gave us, you will find that they are practically identical. They also arrived at a very similar list of cures, or ways to end suffering. I think this is very important. When two sublime teachers with no cultural or historic or personal connection arrive at the same truths, we should take note. They each walked, followed, and created their own unique paths, yet both ended up in the same exalted state.

Something else about these two teachers is also amazing to me. They both used the same metaphor to describe the work we need to do on the level of consciousness. They both used the same analogy to describe the process and the practice. They talked about a "perfect gem," a "flawless jewel."

Not only did they arrive at the same insights and offer the same solutions, they even used the same analogy to describe the inner work! What are the odds of that? They each said that consciousness must be like "a pure flawless diamond." And they said that our consciousness needs to be purified to that extent. Then and only then can it lead to an awakening. As long as our consciousness is dull or controlled by ego, as long as it is full of waves and particles, as long as it is pushed and pulled, or influenced by fear, anger, desire, and so on, it cannot be trusted.

I use the analogy of a fun house mirror. You know the kind that when you stand in front of them make you look tall and skinny with a little pin head, or short and fat with a big old butt! Imagine someone standing there and crying, believing that what they were seeing was real or true. You would laugh at them. You would say: "Don't be silly. That's not how you look. That's not who you are! What you are seeing is the effect of a warped mirror." That is the problem we have with our consciousness.

We look out at the world, or we look at ourselves, we see suffering, limitation, disease, or negativity. But maybe we are not seeing reality at all. Maybe what we see is due to our warped consciousness. That's why we need to do our inner work. That's why we need to quiet and clear our minds; that's why we need to deepen our awareness, to raise and expand our consciousness. And breathwork is a perfect way to do that.

I believe that the Buddha and Patanjali would agree with me here. According to their teachings, they seemed to agree with each other on just about everything. Everything, that is, except one thing. It could be a difference in personal philosophy, or it may simply be a language problem. Maybe they were trying to put something into words that words cannot capture.

My two spiritual buddies seemed to disagree about these two concepts: "consciousness" and "awareness." We tend to think of them as pretty much synonymous, and in fact, the Buddha said they were one and the same, no different. But Patanjali said that they were anything but the same. To him, they could not be more different.

To understand the difference, we can use the analogy of a TV set or a movie screen. Everything that happens on the screen is what we could call the realm of "consciousness." But a TV or a movie screen cannot watch itself. This requires a separate "awareness," something external to or apart from consciousness. Patanjali taught that consciousness was subject to the same laws and dynamics as everything else in nature. Awareness, on the other hand, was not. It was utterly free and not bound in any way to the forces and dynamics and laws that control everything else in nature and the phenomenal world. And this awareness, he said, is who we really are.

I tend to agree because breathwork—spiritual breathing—tends to open us to a direct experience of that state of pure awareness, to that "real true self." In the Song of Solomon, we find these beautiful words: "Breathing restores me to my exact self."

The promise of breathwork—here I'll use the term "breath mastery"—is that it can lead you to a place deep within, to an original, essential being that has never been touched or affected in any way by anything that has happened to you in this world. It is always already pure, still, innocent, and infinitely powerful. Nothing can affect it. Nothing can influence it. Nothing can disturb it in any way: not pain, not fatigue, not fear, not trauma, not love. Nothing, no one, not even you, can influence this place of pure awareness.

It is like a space from which everything arises or occurs. The space doesn't care what fills it: a saint, a sinner, a chair, a flower, my body, or the MacBook on my lap. The space is just a space. This spaciousness is the "exact self" that is referred to in the Song of Solomon and it is that unconditional awareness that Patanjali talked about.

Spiritual breathing is meant to awaken us to this space of pure awareness. We realize that as one of my early teachers said, "I am always already free." We realize that "nothing is happening to me, it is just happening." Breathwork teaches us that everything that happens in life is happening for us, not to us.

We learn in breathwork that we don't need to do anything about what happens in us. We don't have to judge it or understand it, or fix it, or control it. We don't have to resist or manage or change anything about it. We can simply let what is be as it is. We can let ourselves and everything be just as it is. We don't need to resist, judge, attach to anything. In fact, when we stop resisting, attaching, judging, reacting, this space of pure awareness opens up in us, or we open up to it, and we wake up free and at home for the first time to our real true self, to our own infinite eternal being.

Returning to water and consciousness: every thought, every feeling or sensation, every emotion, is another wave or a particle in consciousness. It is like a fun house mirror, and you can't trust it. Only when our consciousness is still and pure can we see through it to what is really real, and only then can we can see what's reflected in it, who we really are. I think that is the real work, the highest purpose of breathwork.

It seems to me that Jesus was also kin to the Buddha and Patanjali. He taught the power of love. He called love the first law of life. To me, love is that space of pure awareness and unmoving presence: love's what's left open and inviting when we let go of all our "stuff" or when it all falls away. We know that Jesus spoke Aramaic, and that most of the original Aramaic language texts have been lost or destroyed over time. I am told that many of the original writings that still exist are in private collections, or locked up somewhere, maybe in the basement of the Vatican. Or maybe that is just a rumor. In any case, I think it is safe to assume that much has been lost in the translation of Jesus' teachings, and some very important things have been twisted, corrupted, deliberately hidden, or simply misunderstood.

For example, I learned from Michael Ryce, the author of *Why Is This Happening to Me, Again?*, that the word "sin" in the Aramaic language is *kata*, which is the word Jesus used when he referred to what we now all call and understand as "sin." Back in Jesus' day, the word "kata" was used in archery, and when an archer missed the mark, the judge would shout *"Kata!"* which simply means "You missed the mark!"[15]

Think about that: when Jesus said that someone had sinned, he was saying that they simply missed the mark. Nothing to do with evil. There is no need for fire and hell and brimstone; all that is required is to adjust our sights.

There is also an expression in the Aramaic language that can be found in no other language. And it is said that Jesus used this expression: "A mind without love is stupid." No wonder He said that love was the first law of life!

The point is that we suffer from the same problem. We are missing the mark, we are missing the point. It's not about sin, punishment, or wrongdoing. It's about the dimension of love. Without love we are blind. Without love we are deaf. Without love we are stupid. Without love we are dumb and numb to the truth of our being, to the truth of life and reality.

The Dimension of Love

Breathwork—spiritual breathing—awakens the dimension of love in us. If I look at the world without eyes of love, I will not see what is really there. If I look at you without eyes of love, I will not see who you really are. If I look at myself without eyes of love, I will not see who I am. This love is very important in breathwork. We need to meet and greet everything we encounter on our inner journey with love. And that love can be expressed perfectly with the breath by opening and expanding, and by relaxing and letting go.

Love shines through when we let go of fear, control, judgments, resistance, and attachments. Love is a space of pure awareness and presence. It is what is left when everything else falls away. Wanting is not loving. Needing is not loving. Expecting or demanding is not loving. Thinking is not loving. Doing is not loving. Well, of course love is in and around all these things, and it can be expressed through them, but . . . And that's a big but!

We all have a biocomputer, what Michael Hewitt-Gleeson, of the School of Thinking and the author of *Software for Your Brain*, calls our "neck-top computer." It has hardware and software, and comes loaded with an operating system. Some of the hardware, some of those programs, and the operating system are quite old and need to be upgraded. Dr. Gleeson talks about Socrates, Aristotle, and Plato; he calls them the "original hackers"—thinking hackers. They created and installed software programs that are still running in our brains today.[16]

Gleeson talks about the "Plato Virus." This virus infects brain users all over the planet, and it is based on the concept of "absolute truth." We forget, he says, that these are just concepts, and a mind that is dominated by this way of thinking gets bogged down. This right-wrong, good-bad, us-them way of thinking has been used to initiate and justify every war and every form of violence in the world for more than two thousand years. It is a useful way of thinking, and yet it represents only one type of thinking.

The concept of good and bad is divisive. It is violent. It may be violence of thought, but it is violence nonetheless. Gleeson offers an upgrade to this ancient software program. Instead of "good and bad," he suggests "good and better." Feel that: "Good . . . Bad." "Good . . . Bad." Breathe, and really feel it. Imagine yourself as a small child hearing those words, and feeling the energy of them. Now try the upgrade: "Good . . . Better." "Good . . . . Better." How does that feel? More loving, right?

What can we accomplish with good and bad that we can't accomplish with good and better? Do we really need good and bad? Is it so important to spend so much energy teaching our children this concept? Most people would probably say: "Of course! What would the world be like if we didn't teach our children the difference between good and bad?" I say it would be heaven on earth. Why do we think that children cannot find their way if we just give them freedom and keep them safe? On one level, I think the worst thing we can say to a child is "Be good!" They are already good! And if they "try" to be good, they become unnatural. Maybe we are training out of our children the very things we are ourselves are trying to reconnect with, because they were trained out of us.

One thing is for sure: when we do breathwork or any inner work, we need to leave that "good-bad, right-wrong" way of thinking at the door. When we take an inner journey, when we approach our inner child, it works best to be free of that divisive way of thinking, otherwise we will do violence on our inner child. What supports our inner journey is to be in our heart when we do breathwork.

❀ BREATHE NOW: HEART-CENTERED MEDITATION

Focus on your heart center. Let your attention drop down out of your head and allow it to settle into the center of your chest. Bring full focused awareness to this place where love resides in you. Someone once said that this could be the longest journey we ever need to make: the twelve inches from our head to our heart.

I like to say that it is no coincidence that the lungs are wrapped around the heart. Maybe the lungs are the wings we need to let our hearts soar! As you open and expand your chest, you create space for the heart to naturally open. Give yourself that experience: use the inhale to create more room, more space in yourself, spaciousness around your heart.

With each slow, full conscious in-breath, meditate on the expansion from side to side, front to back, top to bottom. Let your whole body breathe, with the heart as the center of your experience. No hurry. Focus. Feel.

Imagine breathing into the heart, from the heart, with the heart. Focus on the natural feelings and emotions that resonate in the heart and radiate from it: love, peace, compassion, gratitude . . . Generate the energy of those feelings as you breathe. Fill yourself with these feelings and this energy as you breathe. Send this energy to every cell of your body.

And then on the exhale, allow that energy to radiate out through the pores of your skin, like rays of the sun—those rays, that breath, carrying your heartfelt intentions out in all directions, to everything and everyone. With this meditation, you become a source, a generator, a channel of love energy, and you are the first fortunate recipient of it.

Every day, tens of thousands of Buddhist monks face the four directions of the compass and send peaceful vibrations out into the world. They are praying that all beings be peaceful, that all beings be free from suffering. I think they are making a difference. I believe that we can do our part to compensate for all the ignorance and negative energy in the world by doing this. I am convinced that a heartfelt intention, powered by the breath, can create miracles.

Are you getting the hang of it? Begin to practice this spiritual breathing technique and look for the unfolding of an inner knowing as you begin to realize that every breath is a prayer, and every breath as a blessing.

Everyday Breathing

One of the main things we focus on in breathwork, and one of the main points that we stress at all the seminars, is the importance of putting and keeping ourselves in a positive state. Tony Robbins calls it "a beautiful emotional state," and Barnet Bain calls it "the most amazing feeling." I experience it as a spiritual state.

I am sure that you have had this experience: for some reason or for no reason, you find yourself in a bad mood. Because of that, it seems that everything gets to you; little things that don't usually bother you or bother you very little cause major upsets. Even things that you would usually enjoy, you can't because of the "icky" state that you are in. On the other hand, there are times when for some reason or for no reason at all, you feel very good. In fact, you feel so good that things that usually bother you don't bother you at all. This is due to the state that you are in.

In the practice of spiritual breathing, we make creating or moving into a beautiful state the focus, the priority. The following exercises and meditations are meant to do just that, to put you into the most beautiful and resourceful states. I suggest that you put as much enjoyment into the next few practices as you can, because it is when we are in these beautiful spiritual states that we are able to access the best and the highest in ourselves.

Compassion and Forgiveness

These are feeling states and heart states. The shortcut to regaining them when lost is to focus on our heart and to breathe with a soft gentle quality that combines strength and peace. Imagine a baby who has been teething, cranky, uncomfortable, crying, unable to sleep. Finally, the baby finds relief and is sleeping peacefully. Now you have to pick up the baby and carry her to bed without waking her. How would you handle her? Approach the breath that way: like a sensitive, delicate child.

One of the secrets of breathwork is to put certain conscious qualities into the breath, into the way we breathe. What does compassion feel like? How would a person who is feeling great compassion breathe? Breathe that way. What does it feel like to forgive someone? How does it feel to be forgiven? How would a person who truly forgives or who experiences genuine forgiveness breathe?

There is no right answer waiting to be discovered. You are being called to be it. Focus on the feelings of compassion and forgiveness and use your breath to give them form and expression.

Connecting

We are all sucking off the same bubble of air that surrounds this planet. And so the breath already connects us to everyone and everything whether we are aware of it or not. Bring that feeling of connection alive in yourself. Learn to use the breath to wake yourself up to an experience of it. When you watch a sunset, don't just take it in with your eyes, take it in with the breath. When you are listening to something or someone, draw the energy of what you hear into you with the breath. When you touch something, take in the feeling of it with the breath. Everything is energy, and once we are in touch with the energy in the breath, we can get in touch with everything.

Feel Amazing

Think of a time when you felt amazing, when everything was wonderful, when you were extremely happy, when you felt truly and totally alive, open, inspired, connected. Maybe you were falling in love. Maybe you were looking into the eyes of your infant. Perhaps drinking in a sunset, making a perfect tennis shot, baking a perfect batch of cookies, making a great presentation, or closing a successful business deal. Maybe you were preparing for a holiday or enjoying a celebration. Or maybe you were serving someone, making a difference in the world or in someone's life, or making a contribution to something greater than yourself.

When you have that memory in mind, imagine it in present time. Step into it as if it is happening right now. And feel it fully. What is the quality of that experience? The feeling? Start to use every breath to make that feeling more alive in you. Generate the feeling, feed and fuel it with the inhale. Use the exhale to relax into it and enjoy it. Be very Zen-like. Keep your focus moment to moment, breath by breath, on this most amazing feeling.

De-Reflexive Breathing

When you physically inhale, mentally exhale. When you physically exhale, mentally inhale. That sums up a spiritual breathing technique called De-reflexive Breathing. It is also called Krishna's kriya yoga. There is more to it than that, but getting the hang of this main piece of it is big!

As you breathe, imagine that air and light are traveling along the same path at the same time but in opposite directions. Some people like to use their hands to represent the light. As we breathe air in, light moves out and away from us; and as we breathe air out, light flows in and toward us.

This meditation is meant to dissolve the illusion of separateness and to break the habit of body identification. It is meant to help us merge with the energy that fills and surrounds everything and everyone. As a friend once told me, everything in the universe has consciousness, and when we get too fixated on our own consciousness, we get out of balance with the rest of the universe.

Three Waves of Peace, Love, Joy

Focus on your heart and generate the energy of love and peace and joy as you breathe in. Fill yourself with it, and then release this energy out into the world with your exhale. Let each breath be like a wave. As when a stone is thrown into a pool of water, that circular wave that goes out in all directions.

Take three long inhales and three big sighs of relief as you focus on your heart. Feel yourself filling with love, peace, and joy, and then send that energy out into the world, like a flower releasing its fragrance. A heartfelt intention powered by the breath can do magic in the world.

Spiritual Vacuum Cleaner

This is an advanced meditation for the daring of heart. Breathe all the negative energy of the world into your heart and let the heart transform it into positive energy. Breathe in pain, breathe out pleasure. Breathe in fear, breathe out safety. Breathe in hate, breathe out love. The heart is a transformer. Trust it. Make use of it. Breathe in sadness, breathe out gratitude. Breathe from your heart.

The energy does not linger in you. It passes through without slowing down. Be like a child: innocent. Believe that the heart can magically and instantly transform any energy into love and joy and peace. The heart knows how to do this. With our heart, we can see the divinity in everyone. With our heart, we can see the perfection in everything. This is not a head thing. It is a feeling thing. It is a heartfelt creative thing.

5

BREATHING SUCCESS IN LIFE, LOVE, BUSINESS, AND BEYOND

If you can do something with the breath, you will attain the source of life. If you can do something with the breath, you can transcend time and space. If you can do something with the breath, you will be in the world and also beyond it.

— *THE BOOK OF SECRETS,* **OSHO**

In the fall of 1969 when I was training as an X-ray technician I saw an invitation on the bulletin board to learn cardiopulmonary resuscitation (CPR). I signed up without the slightest thought. The desire to learn to breathe life into another human being was instant, automatic, and irresistible. I couldn't believe it when I showed up for the course and discovered that I was the only one from my department attending.

A few weeks later, I was sent to the intensive care unit to take a routine portable chest X-ray. John, I learned later, was a baseball talent scout. As soon as I walked into the room I felt something was not right.

I leaned in as closely as I could to him, carefully looking, listening, and feeling. He was not breathing! Just then, the *beep, beep, beep* coming from his cardiac monitor turned into a long, steady *beeeeeeeeep*. His heart stopped cold, and in that moment, mine began to race. I checked his pulse. Sure enough: nothing! I peeled open his eyelids: his pupils were fixed and dilated. He was clinically dead.

I jumped into action and did everything by the book, exactly as I was instructed and had practiced in class. I threw his pillow onto the floor behind me. I tilted his head back, pinched his nose, covered his mouth with mine, and blew a big breath into him. I watched his chest fill, and then watched and listened as his chest collapsed and the air escaped.

I blew another big breath into him then yelled for help. I positioned my hands over his sternum just as I had been taught and did five quick heart compressions. Nurses and doctors began arriving, but had trouble getting themselves and the crash cart into the room because my X-ray machine was blocking the door.

The bed was too soft, his whole body was giving in under the pressure of my hands, and I was worried that the heart compressions were not being effective. I heard myself shout: "We need a backboard! Someone get a backboard!" Was that my voice? It was two octaves higher than normal. I realized that to help him, the first thing I needed to do was to relax and take a breath for myself.

A couple of people on the team quickly slid the backboard under him, and I blew two more big breaths into him. As I started another series of compressions, I felt more confident. A nurse leaned in with an Ambu bag (a manual resuscitator) to take over the ventilations.

One of the doctors was getting in position beside me, preparing to take over the manual compressions, when suddenly John came alive with a jolt. His eyes shot open. He looked startled, afraid for a moment, but then extremely peaceful. Just like that, he began to breathe on his own. Someone checked and said: "Good strong pulse." It was over almost as soon as it had begun.

Most of the ICU team went back to what they were doing, with no fanfare whatsoever. To them, I suppose it was business as usual, just another day at the office. But I wanted to jump up and down and shout. This was a freaking miracle! A few minutes ago the man had been clinically dead, and now he was alive and breathing again. I wanted to celebrate. I wanted to cry. I needed to hug somebody.

Two of the nurses had stayed in the room. With calm and meticulous care, they got all of his tubes and wires back in order. One of them asked him: "How are you feeling?" He didn't answer. Energy from the adrenaline as well as from the joy was vibrating in me and streaming through me. I was high as kite and shaking like a leaf.

I stood in the doorway leaning on my X-ray machine, feeling elated, watching and listening to John's breathing. When the nurses were done, I did what I was sent there to do: I took his X-ray, and pretended that it was just another day at the office for me too. But truly it was the most amazing and wonderful day of my life. I was hooked on the miracle of breath!

After that first experience, I had the opportunity to resuscitate more than a dozen people over the next ten years. When you love what you do, life gives you lots of opportunities to do it! And I also trained several thousand other people to perform CPR, a skill definitely worth having and sharing!

• • •

The breath is in many ways our closest friend and helper in life; it is our constant companion from birth to rebirth. It faithfully supports us in everything we do whether or not we are aware of it, and whether or not we appreciate it. Our breath in many ways is like the canary in the coal mine. Do you know this story?

In the old days, coal miners often died when pockets of poisonous gases were uncovered in the mining process. These gases were often odorless and tasteless, so they learned to bring a canary down into the mines with them. Because the bird was more sensitive than the men, it would succumb to the deadly gases before the miners were even aware of it. Those birds saved countless lives. And our breath is like this canary: it responds to things that we are not conscious or aware of.

I've always been fascinated by a particular biorhythm, a natural phenomenon that the ancients believed was so important that an entire branch of yoga, called swara yoga, evolved around it. Did you know your breath swings back and forth like a pendulum between your left and right nostrils about every hour or so, and it has been doing this since the day you were born?

Check it out now. Close one nostril and breathe in and out through the opposite one; then switch and breathe in and out through the other. Which nostril feels more open? Which feels more constricted? Check it again after a while, and you will probably find that it has changed. There are also times when the nostrils are equally open and balanced.

This right and left nostril dominance is no doubt connected to left- and right-brain activity, and you can set your watch by it. This rhythm also happens to be one of the first rhythms to be disturbed when something in us goes out of balance, and when illness creeps in. The swara yogis developed various exercises and techniques to influence this rhythm, to adjust and rebalance it when necessary.

What's more, the yogis discovered that this rhythm is related to aspects of life far beyond the body—things like sun and moon and planetary cycles and astrology. They scheduled mental and physical activities such as waking and sleeping, bathing and eating, working and meditating according to this rhythm. They considered it when deciding to focus on a math problem and when to write poetry. They turned to it to know when to ask a favor of the king, when to go into battle, when to pray, when to work in the garden, and when to make love.

For more than a year, I was obsessed with this yogic practice. I kept a small crescent-shaped mirror in my pocket, and dozens of times each day, I would take it out, put it under my nose, and breathe onto it. I would study the size and shape of the two moist clouds that appeared, noting the time of day, my general mood, where I was, what I was doing, who was with me, and what was happening. I learned a lot about myself and others, about life and the world, and the breath and breathing.

I am not suggesting that you need to be quite that fanatical— okay, wait, maybe I am! No, really, what I am saying is that there are lots of things related to the breath that we have not discovered or explored, and that breathing is related to every level of our being, that it holds many mysteries, and that breathwork can be used to improve every area of our lives.

Breathing to the Symphony of Life

I loved my daily visits to the Metropol Hotel in Moscow in the early nineties, when I was leading seminars. The Russians called what I did "free breathing," and I happened to be teaching for free, so the term was perfect. I liked the hotel because I could get out of the cold, read English-language newspapers, and enjoy a hot coffee in the lobby bar or restaurant. I would often drop in just to use the bathroom: it was clean and warm and they had American-style toilet paper rather than old newspapers or the local brand that literally had wood chips in it! I visited the hotel so often that everyone assumed I lived there. It got to the point where I could go up to the desk and request a courtesy car—basically a free taxi service!

All warmed up and caught up on the news, I walked out to the street one day and decided to wander through a section of the city center I had not explored. I noticed people carrying musical instruments, walking briskly, coming from different directions, and all converging on one location. I followed them into a small auditorium and sat in the back of the hall watching them tune up and settle down. I don't remember his name, but soon the most famous conductor in Russia at the time appeared. Everyone was quite excited to have the opportunity to rehearse with him.

The music they made gave me goose bumps. I played with my breath, following along, keeping the rhythm, and varying the intensity of my inhales and exhales depending on the mood or speed of the music. I think that I never really appreciated classical music until that day. You see, I grew up loving rock and roll, folk, and pop music.

My mind drifted back to my childhood and music appreciation class in Catholic school. The nuns would play classical pieces, and we kids would all chuckle or be bored to tears. It all sounded the same to us: just a bunch of violins—one big noise. However, as I watched and listened that day, I was struck by the details that the conductor was able to catch.

There were more than forty violinists, and if just one of them was a moment too soon or a moment too late with their note, he would catch it. For me, if five of those violinists had stayed home that day, I would not even have noticed the difference. And with a hundred musicians all playing together, one flute player was too quiet or too loud, the conductor would stop and scold them. Heck, I didn't even know there was a flute player in the band. I began to understand how much more that conductor could appreciate music than me.

Breathing is like that: it's like listening to a symphony orchestra. The average person thinks: "Breathe in, breathe out. What's the big deal?" I will tell you. There are points in the breathing that you have never observed, and those points, as the spiritual teacher Osho once said, are like doors to a new consciousness, a new reality. But they are very subtle.

I invite you to become the master of your instrument and the conductor of your orchestra. When you do—when you begin to catch the subtleties, the details, the power, the beauty—you too can begin to perform and accomplish the most remarkable things in life. When you tune in to the breath and open to it, the breath opens and tunes in to you.

When you learn to appreciate and master your breath, life opens up to you in ways that the average person can only dream of, or cannot even imagine.

Most people can talk and sing and dance, throw a ball, use a pen or a paintbrush, or cook a meal, but some people find a way through practice and devotion of raising these things to the level of an art. Breathing is like that. We all breathe, but we can learn to breathe in ways that lead to the most powerful and beautiful states and abilities. We can develop a relationship to the breath that allows us to become spiritual maestros. With this in mind, let's play with another exercise.

✳ BREATHE NOW: LISTENING MEDITATION

Play a couple of your favorite pieces of music. Maybe use headphones. As you are listening to the music, begin to take in the music with your breath. Breathe in rhythm to it. Synchronize the movement of your breath with the movement of the music. Play with your breath while you listen. Vary the speed and volume and intensity of your breathing as the pace and rhythm and mood of the music changes.

Make breath sounds (on both the inhale and the exhale). Put passion and enthusiasm into the breathing as you listen and take part in the performance. Express with your breath the feelings that the music awakens in you.

Use the breathing to disappear into the music. Have fun! Experiment. You may find a whole new level of enjoyment and appreciation of music. And you will be developing your breathing mechanism in the process, giving it more range and flexibility. Use your favorite music to expand your breathing repertoire.

The Key to Ultimate Transformation

It's one thing to be in charge of our process. It's one thing to be using the breath to generate love, peace, and joy; to work with the healing, creative, and restorative powers of the breath. It's quite another to be lifted up by the breath itself and taken on a magnificent journey.

The real miracle of the breath occurs only when we learn how to turn it on, fire it up, and set it free to do its work in us; when we can let it take over our very being, when we can surrender to it while it shakes all the fear and stress and tension from the cells of our body, like a dog shakes off water.

We attain the highest states when we can, as the Quakers say, open all the doors and windows of our being and let the power of the Holy Spirit blow through. The Holy Spirit is the breath! If you are worried about the wind knocking over all the knickknacks on your shelves, if you insist on holding on to your old limiting beliefs about who you are or what is possible, then you will consciously and unconsciously fight the full, free flow of the breath. Thus you can expect that spirit will sit quietly and lovingly at your door waiting until you are "ready."

I hope something in this book triggers that readiness, because without it, the greatest gifts of the spirit, of the breath, can never be received. When a spiritual seeker is ready, the next book they pick up will have the answer, the next teacher they meet will show them the way, the next technique they practice will cause a breakthrough. It really has very little to do with the book, or the teacher, or the technique: it has everything to do with readiness. With that readiness, even something as simple and natural as the breath will set you free and fulfill your heart's eternal desire.

Guiding Life Principles

My path and breathing program, called Breath Mastery, brings all these tools and techniques, methods, and strategies together for the purpose of self-mastery. This is the essence and the purpose of the practice, and it represents the focus of my work.

To gain the ultimate promise of Breath Mastery we need to develop a certain faith in ourselves. We need to build a certain trust in our natural divinity. We are called to nurture a sense of oneness with all existence, and an appreciation for the perfection of life. We must be willing to be aware and at ease with whatever is, as it is, moment to moment. And it requires a heartfelt intention to hold a space of conscious, active, all-inclusive, unconditional love. It's a grand task to be sure, and in a way, it cannot be taught, it can only be caught.

Breathing patterns are like fingerprints: unique to each of us. Your breathing pattern says a lot about you, about your relationship to yourself, to your body, and to life. Every physiological, emotional, and psychological state has a corresponding or associated breathing pattern. The way you breathe when you are angry and upset is different from the way you breathe when you are peaceful and calm. The way you breathe when you're afraid or in pain is different from the way you breathe when you're feeling comfort and pleasure.

When your state changes, your breathing pattern changes. And it's a two-way street: when you change your breathing, you change your state. And therein lays the transformational power and the healing potential of breathwork.

Every time you "take over" the breathing you are reprogramming your "autopilot." If fear, guilt, anger, shame, or confusion causes your breathing to change, you can regain your balance and return to a resourceful state by controlling your breath. When your breathing is blocked or chaotic, rushed or held, it produces or aggravates various psychological and emotional conditions. Certain thoughts tend to produce certain feelings, and vice versa. That's why it's important to generate wonderful, positive, bright, loving thoughts and feelings when you breathe. Whatever thoughts and feelings you focus on while you breathe, you can be sure that the breath is giving life to them. So be careful what you think about when you breathe!

The following guiding principles or active forces are also choices and states of consciousness. They reflect my spiritual commitment in life and to this work. They represent both the process and the path of Breath Mastery:

Oneness and wholeness
Energy and aliveness
Freedom and safety
Peace and power
Love and light
Health and happiness
Rhythm and balance
Circles and cycles
Forgiveness and gratitude

If you can incorporate these guiding principles into your breathing, make them your focus as you breathe, honor and commit to supporting them, your rewards will be endless.

6

TWENTY-ONE-DAY BREATH MASTERY CHALLENGE

I invite you to take a three-week journey with me into the power and potential of breathwork. Each day we will explore a different breathing exercise, technique, or meditation. The course is designed to give you a broad and solid foundation and to help you develop the knowledge and skills you need to master your breath as a tool for health, growth, and change in body, mind, and spirit.

Do your best to follow the minimum practice formula: 10 + 10 + (10 x 2). That means ten minutes in the morning, ten minutes at night, and ten times during the day for two minutes. Most people have no problem fitting an extra ten minutes into their morning and evening rituals. The real challenge is getting into the habit of stopping about once every hour throughout the day to do two minutes of Conscious Breathing practice. Don't beat yourself up if you can't hold to the schedule, just do your best to work in as many of these mini sessions as you can. I think you will find that the benefits you get from this protocol will motivate you to do much more.

You may want to spend more time on some of the exercises and techniques, and you may even want to stick with an especially interesting, enjoyable, or challenging exercise for several days. That's perfectly okay. Move through the lessons at your own pace, but don't skip over any of them or give any of them less attention just because they seem easy or simple. Give each lesson your full attention and focus.

If you want to accelerate your progress or deepen your practice, then dedicate twenty minutes in the morning and twenty minutes at night instead of ten, or slip in a ten- or twenty-minute midday training/practice session on top of the ten two-minute sessions.

There is another practice option for those who cannot manage to do ten two-minute sessions through the day—call it a Plan B—which is three times per day for five, ten, or twenty minutes each time. As you can see, the bare minimum is three five-minute practice sessions each day. If you choose this option, you will definitely experience many benefits, but I hope you will choose something more than the absolute minimum—especially if you are interested in breath mastery; or if you would like to use the breath to heal or improve some physical, emotional, or psychological issue or challenge; or if your goal is optimum health, peak performance, or ultimate potential.

Whatever you decide, and whatever you do, make sure to note it in your breathing diary or breathwork journal. Jot down what you practiced and what you felt, what happened, what you learned or realized. At the end of the course, go back over the exercises and select the ones you really liked and go deeper into the practice of them. You may also choose to combine several exercises to create your own unique practice.

Note: Unless specified as part of the exercise, you can breathe through your nose or your mouth—whatever feels easy, interesting, or comfortable. Unless the particular exercise calls for mouth or nose breathing, do yourself a favor and experiment with both.

One more note: A couple of the advanced techniques and therapeutic practices can require up to an hour or more of continuous engagement. These techniques are noted and are best done with a breathing buddy, a qualified coach, or a certified breathworker (in person or via Skype).

If you would like my support, become a member of my Breath Mastery Inner Circle. All the information is at www.breathmastery.com. To find a breathwork coach near you, contact office@breathmastery.com.

Day One: Breath Watching

Breath mastery starts with Breath Awareness. In order to get the full benefits of breathwork, you'll need to develop a very conscious and intimate relationship with your breath.

The main thing about the practice of Breath Awareness is that you are not doing the breathing. You are not breathing in any particular way: you are allowing the breath to come and go by itself while you are simply an impartial observer, a detached witness. This is a mindfulness practice, also called breath watching.

Observe your breathing right now. Ten minutes is good; twenty minutes is better. Commit to making this a regular daily practice.

If the breath moves through your nose, focus your attention on the feelings and sensations in your nostrils as the air passes in and out. If you are breathing through your mouth, notice the feelings and sensations of the air as it passes over your lips and tongue. You can also focus on the feelings and sensations of movement in your chest or belly as the breath comes and goes.

If your mind wanders (and it will), if you get caught up in thinking, or if something else pulls your attention away from the breath or distracts you from it, simply place your attention back on the breath as soon as you can. Focus totally on the next breath. Reward yourself by taking a particularly pleasurable breath that energizes and relaxes you.

Start to develop the habit of tuning in to your breathing at various times and during various activities. For example, notice how you breathe while you walk, work, and lift things. Notice your breathing during personal interactions with others.

Also begin to notice how other people breathe. Pay attention to the breathing of the people you live with, work with, and play with. Pay attention to how they breathe when they speak, move, strain, complain, and celebrate, when they are angry, nervous, embarrassed, and so on. Paying attention to other people's breathing will make you more conscious of your own.

Day Two: Yawning and Sighing

Today, we move from the passive practice of Breath Awareness to the active practice of Conscious Breathing. However, in order to start off properly, we are going to take our cue from nature and start with two natural reflexes or breathing responses: yawning and sighing.

A sigh is made up of an inhale that is twice as big as usual or normal followed by a long, relaxing exhale. The key to this exercise is to make your inhale twice as big or deep or full as a normal-sized inhale. It's like adding one inhale on top of the other. You are to create an extra stretch or expansion on the inhale, which will automatically trigger a bigger or longer exhale than usual. This natural breath done consciously will both energize and relax you.

If you are like most people, you are already taking a sigh about every five minutes, or twelve times per hour. Nature makes you do this in order to inflate all the alveoli, to keep your lungs healthy and maintain your respiratory capacity. If you are practicing Breath Awareness, you will begin to catch these unconscious, automatic sighs when they happen. When you do, I suggest that you cooperate with them: follow them up with another deliberate sigh. Double down on nature!

Practice an expanded inhale and a luxurious sigh of relief right now. Exaggerate it. Make it dramatic. Be theatrical! When you breathe in, get the sense of adding one inhale on top of the other, adding an extra stretch to the inhale, and then when you let the exhale go, deliberately relax. Use the exhale to consciously release any physical tension from your jaw, neck, and shoulders.

Taking a couple of these breaths may trigger a yawn. If not, go ahead and trigger one on purpose. Wiggle your jaw and do something in the upper part of your throat as you inhale to deliberately activate the yawning reflex. And just as you did with the sigh of relief, exaggerate it. Make it dramatic. Make it a full-body experience. Add enjoyable sounds and pleasurable stretching to the yawn.

And now here is the real key: Combine a yawn and a sigh. When giving yourself a big, conscious sigh of relief, deliberately trigger the yawning reflex. And when you are yawning, deliberately give yourself a big, expansive inhale and a luxurious sigh of relief.

Trigger the yawning reflex, and as you do, breathe big, expanded inhales and big sighs of relief. Mix yawning and sighing. Practice this right now for the next five or ten minutes. Stretch and move and make sounds as you practice. Make it a full-body experience. Observe the effect it has on your energy, your mood, and your mental state.

Plug this exercise into your daily practice protocol 10 + 10 + (10 x 2). Use it when completing one activity or when you are about to begin another. Use it to cool your brain and to provide a healthy stretch to your lungs. Use it to feel more awake and relaxed. Do it just because it feels good and because it's good for you.

Have fun with it, and have fun with the reactions you are sure to get from the people around you when you do it. This exercise should make for some very interesting journal entries!

Day Three: Diaphragmatic Breathing or "Belly Breathing"

Many people have the habit of breathing shallow breaths high in their chest. This pattern can activate the fight-or-flight reflex or a stress reaction; it tends to keep us anxious or on the edge of irritation and anxiety. Today, we want to practice the opposite of that. We want to apply the general rule for antistress, anti-anxiety: breathe low and slow.

Slow, diaphragmatic breathing is a fundamental key to optimum health and peak performance, so you need to master it at all costs. It needs to become second nature.

Many men, when they take in a deep breath, focus only on puffing up their chests. And many women, concerned about their appearance, tend to hold their bellies in when they breathe. We need to breathe down into an area called the *dan tien* or the *hara*. It is the center of gravity in your body, a couple of inches below your navel, midway front to back. Breathing this way needs to become our unconscious, automatic resting pattern.

Right now, put one hand over your belly button and one hand on your upper chest and practice breath watching. Which hand moves most? Which hand moves first? Are you a chest breather or a belly breather? If you are a habitual chest breather, you absolutely must change that pattern. If you are already a natural belly breather, you will benefit greatly by consciously deepening and strengthening that healthy pattern.

Practice it lying on your back with your knees bent and your feet flat on the floor. As you breathe in, arch your lower back; and as you exhale, press your lower back to the floor.

As you are inhaling and arching your lower spine, notice that your pelvis wants to rotate or tilt downward and back (like sticking your butt out). As you exhale and press your lower spine to the floor, notice that your pelvis wants to tilt or rotate upward and forward (like tucking your butt in).

In fact, just by rhythmically moving your spine and pelvis this way with each breath, your body will naturally "pump" air in and out. Get a sense of this pumping action. In addition to supporting healthy breathing, this exercise is good for loosening up and strengthening your lower back.

Another way to train in diaphragmatic breathing is to put a book or some other object, like a small sandbag, on your belly. When you inhale, lift the book up with your breath. When you exhale, let the book settle down again. Without any props, simply breathe slowly and consciously, and as you breathe in, let your belly pop out. As you breathe out, pull your belly button in toward your spine. This is diaphragmatic or belly breathing.

While sitting, place your hands over your belly button, interlacing your fingers very lightly. When you inhale, your hands and fingers should move apart. When you exhale, your hands and fingers should come together again.

When standing, place your hands on each side of your waist, above your hip bones, fingers toward the front and thumbs toward the back. When you exhale, squeeze your hands in toward your midline and squeeze your fingers together. When you inhale, you should feel the breath pushing your hands apart and spreading your fingers open.

To improve your diaphragmatic breathing, practice applying more pressure with your hands and fingers and inhaling against this pressure.

Day Four: The Therapeutic Zone

Getting comfortable with a rate of six breaths per minute is extremely therapeutic. Today, you want to focus on that pattern. If six breaths per minute is too difficult, then aim for eight or ten. If six is easy, aim for four or five.

Six breaths per minute means a five-second inhale and a five-second exhale, with only a slight momentary transition between the inhale and the exhale and between the exhale and the inhale. The breathing is rhythmic and feels continuous and smooth.

In, 2, 3, 4, 5

Out, 2, 3, 4, 5

In, 2, 3, 4, 5

Out, 2, 3, 4, 5

This is a breathing pattern that you can settle into whenever you like. It's a great way to focus the mind and to relax and energize the body. It also increases heart rate variability (HRV), something we discussed at length in chapter 2.

If the four-to-six-breaths-per-minute range is way out of your comfort zone, start with twelve breaths per minute and gradually slow it down. If you run out of breath or you are already full before you've reached the end of your count, just gently hold or pause the breath while you finish counting.

Day Five: Engaging the Exhale

Learning to snap the exhale loose, to release it quickly and completely, is a powerful skill. If you have not learned how to let go of your exhale, don't be surprised if you can't let go of tension or pain, fear or anxiety, or thoughts that keep going around and around in your head: you have not learned the energetic skill of letting go. We can develop this ability by using the breath. Once you learn to let go of the exhale quickly and completely, you will be surprised at what else you can easily let go of.

When you pull in a full inhale, you create internal pressure, and you stretch all the chest muscles. You can then use that pressure and the elastic tendency of your muscles to do the exhale for you. The exhale is reflexive. You don't need to blow or to push; you simply relax and let go and the breath pours out by itself. Try it now. Pull in a big inhale and then snap the exhale loose. Release it. Dump it out. Let it go quickly and completely. Don't control the exhale. Don't let it out slowly. Set the exhale free and allow all the breath to pour out of you as close to all at once as possible—like a balloon popping.

There is a knack to this, and when you catch it, it feels great. And once you know how to engage the exhale, it will help you in those moments when you need to let go on some other level.

Day Six: Linking Movement and Breath

"Lead with the breath." That advice comes from the great dance and breathing teacher Ilsa Middendorf. It also comes from the legendary Mikhail Ryabko, the founder of Systema Russian martial arts. When two totally different teachers from two separate cultures and fields of endeavor arrive at the same insight, we should pay attention.

Every martial artist, boxer, and athlete knows the power of synchronizing movement and breath. Listen to some of the leading tennis players every time they hit the ball. You will find this principle in karate, weight lifting, tai chi, chi kung, and yoga, as well as Taoist and Sufi practices. Today, you are going to begin to make it part of your breathwork practice.

We already touched on this when we focused on diaphragmatic breathing, arching the spine and tilting the pelvis with each breath:

breath moving the body, body moving the breath, body and breath moving together.

This practice can be as simple as opening your hands while you inhale and closing them as you exhale. It could mean opening your arms as if welcoming someone on the inhale and then folding them over your heart on the exhale, or tilting your head back and looking up as you inhale and then tucking your chin in and looking down as you exhale. Another possibility is turning at the waist in one direction as you inhale and twisting in the other direction as you exhale.

Reach up with both arms as if grabbing air on the inhale, then sharply pull your arms down, making fists, with the exhale. Combining the breath and any movement is as much a meditation as it is an exercise.

Breathe in rhythm to your footsteps. There is an entire book called *Breathwalk* by Gurucharan Singh Khalsa and Yogi Bhajan dedicated to this simple, yet powerful practice.[17]

In fact, you can turn the simple act of getting up from a chair into a breathing exercise. Start inhaling a second or two before you start to stand, and continue the inhale until you reach a fully upright position. Then start exhaling a moment or two before you begin lowering yourself back to a sitting position, ending the exhale as you settle all your weight fully onto the chair.

You can combine breathing with push-ups, squats, sit-ups, or any repetitive physical movement. This is your chance to get creative. For example, if you have two flights of stairs to climb at your office, you could inhale while climbing the first flight and exhale while climbing the second flight. Or you could simply inhale as you lift and place your left foot and exhale as you lift and place your right foot.

Today, synchronize your breathing to your movements. Be conscious of your breathing while your body is in action. Let your intuition and your imagination guide you. This is a serious practice, so have fun with it!

A reminder: Let the breath be like the locomotive engine at the head of a train. The engine moves a bit, and then the first car moves forward slightly, followed by the second, then the third, and like that all the way down the line until the whole train is moving. Let your breath be that engine: move it first, and let your body follow. In other words, lead with the breath.

Day Seven: Three Breathing Spaces and the Full Yogic Breath

Consider that you have three breathing spaces: a lower space from the perineum to the belly button; a middle breathing space from the navel to the nipple line; and an upper space from the nipple line to the collarbones.

The full yogic breath is like filling a glass with water: it fills from the bottom up. The full yogic breath fills the entire breathing cavity with each in-breath, and it sends a lovely wave of energy through the body when done smoothly and powerfully.

To make the process even more beneficial and enjoyable, imagine filling yourself with light, love, peace, joy, strength, courage, clarity, health. In other words, focus not only on breathing air, but also on breathing energy (prana, chi, ki).

Do this exercise sitting, either on the floor in the classic cross-legged position or on a chair, spine straight but relaxed. Your chin should be slightly tucked in, the tongue lightly touching the roof of your mouth, where the soft palate meets the hard palate (to close the energetic loop).

1. Send the first part of the in-breath all the way down to your perineum and feel your lower belly expand.

2. Allow the breath to overflow up into the rib cage, breathing into your back and feeling your chest expand from side to side.

3. Fill the upper part of your chest. Feel the collarbones rising up toward the chin. (Don't use your shoulders or tense your neck muscles when you breathe.)

In the beginning you can mentally count: one . . . two . . . three . . . as you fill the lower space, the middle space, and the upper space, each in turn. In time, it all becomes one long, smooth breath with three seamless phases.

Remember that even as you are filling the upper space, the lower space continues to fill and expand. (Don't pull in on the belly as you aim the breath high into the chest.) Give yourself the sense that you are expanding from top to bottom, side to side, and front to back as you breathe in.

When exhaling, release the entire breathing mechanism at once, and feel the top, middle, and lower spaces empty in turn.

Remember that this is a breathing meditation as much as it is a breathing exercise.

Day Eight: Burst Breathing

Breathe in through your nose and out through your mouth. Take little short breaths in and out as fast as you can. The accent is on the inhale.

My teacher, chi kung master Hu Bin, taught this to me in 1985 when I visited Beijing, but he had no specific name for it. I was very happy when I heard Vladimir Vasiliev, author of *Let Every Breath* . . . , refer to this as "burst breathing."

Burst breathing can help you to quickly recover from a painful blow or a sudden shock. You can also use it when you need to quickly rest and recharge yourself while maintaining movement or exerting force or resistance—for example, in grappling or weight lifting.

Burst breathing is a great way to "suck" pain or fatigue from your muscles and vent it from the body. Breathing very short, very quick breaths is a way to loosen up your breathing mechanism. At the same time, you are getting practice at instantly shifting breathing channels: nose, mouth, nose, mouth, nose, mouth

Because the breaths are so short and quick, you don't have time to move a lot of air with each cycle, but try to take in and release as much air as you can with each quick burst. Be very conscious of any tension and unnecessary effort. Ease, efficiency, and economy of effort are important.

Start now: breathe short quick breaths in through the nose and out through the mouth for a few minutes. The focus or accent is on the inhale; the exhale is reflexive. Breathe in this way as quickly as you can, at a smooth, steady pace. If you get all jammed up, if the breathing becomes sticky or chaotic, slow down just enough to do it right and then gradually speed it up again. You should aim for two cycles per second, or 120 breaths per minute. Breathe normally for a minute or so and then do another round of burst breathing.

It's okay to ease off or take a couple of long, slow breaths from time to time as you practice the rapid breathing. This is training. Be patient with yourself, but be persistent.

Day Nine: Box Breathing

Box breathing, also called "square breathing," incorporates breath holding with inhales and exhales. It strengthens mental focus and our powers of concentration. It is a mindfulness practice. It also balances our energy and our nervous systems.

Breathe in for a count of four, hold for a count of four, exhale for a count of four, hold for a count of four. Don't tense your body or lock up your breathing during the holding. It is more like an "open pause."

If you are measuring your count in seconds, you will be breathing at a rate of just under four breaths per minute. But it is not necessary to measure your breaths by the clock. Simply balance all four phases—inhale, hold, exhale, hold—keeping them all equal in length.

This is a great breath exercise to do anytime that you want to be in an energetically balanced or neutral state. It is a good way to prepare for a stressful event or a complex activity. It is not for use during complicated tasks. Plug this exercise into your training protocol today and practice it when standing in line at the bank or when stuck in traffic, or anytime you need to be grounded, focused, alert, and relaxed.

Day Ten: Reverse or Paradoxical Breathing

Today, let's practice a very healthy and powerful Chinese medicinal breathing exercise called "reverse respiration" or "paradoxical breathing." This way of breathing is also practiced in many yoga traditions.

As you recall, normally, when we inhale the diaphragm "moves" downward, causing the belly to pop out, and when we exhale, the diaphragm "rises up" and the belly is drawn inward toward the spine.

With reverse respiration, we reverse this natural movement by deliberately pulling in on the belly while inhaling, and then popping the belly out while exhaling (thus the term "reverse" or "paradoxical").

This way of breathing creates strong intra-abdominal pressures, which in addition to toning the diaphragm and strengthening abdominal muscles helps improve digestive and intestinal problems as well as gynecological conditions. It is also used in chi kung to "pack" chi into the fascia; and it is used in tantric meditations to raise kundalini or draw sexual energy up into the heart. (Kundalini is another name for our life force energy.)

Sometimes this pattern of sucking in the belly as you inflate the chest can become chronic. This creates constant stress, weakens the diaphragm, and creates imbalances and unnecessary wear and tear on the system. For those who have unconsciously adopted this unhealthy pattern, taking conscious control of it with this exercise is the best way to stop it and restore internal balance and natural breathing.

Reverse respiration or paradoxical breathing can be done standing or sitting. It's always a good idea to experiment in different postures and various positions.

Start with the exhale. As you exhale and empty your lungs, blow the breath out either through pursed lips or with a *shush* sound, or through the nose. As you do, deliberately push or pop your belly out.

Then, when you inhale, suck the belly in, pull the belly button toward the spine, and pull up on the perineum, as if you are trying to tuck all your abdominal organs up under your rib cage and high into your chest.

Take your time with this exercise. Focus. Use some muscular effort as you push the belly out during the exhale and suck the belly in during the inhale, but don't force or strain.

After eight or ten rounds or several minutes of reverse breathing, rest and allow the breath to flow naturally in and out by itself, or practice natural diaphragmatic breathing in between rounds.

Day Eleven: Alternate-Nostril Breathing

This is an ancient Conscious Breathing exercise, and it is a basic practice in traditional *pranayama*, the yogic science of breath. The practice of alternate-nostril breathing has an extremely positive effect on your physical, emotional, and mental health. In fact, it is a perfect exercise for getting control of runaway thinking, useless mental chatter, or an out-of-control mind.

Left/right nostril dominance is connected to left/right brain activity, and according to the ancients, it also relates to the sun, moon, and planetary cycles. In general, the left nostril stimulates the right brain and is associated with emotional, musical, visual, calming, cooling, relaxing, eliminating, female, and lunar activities. The right nostril stimulates the left brain and is associated with rational, verbal, warming, energizing, male, and solar activities.

This basic prana yoga exercise involves using the thumb and ring finger of your right hand to alternately block your right and left nostril. Most people like to rest their index and/or middle finger on their forehead between the eyebrows (over the "third eye").

When practicing alternate-nostril breathing, start with the exhale. The idea is to empty your lungs and clear the channel before drawing in a fresh new stream of breath.

Block your right nostril with your right thumb and exhale and inhale one breath through the left nostril. Then switch: block your left nostril with the ring finger of your right hand and exhale and inhale one breath through the right nostril. Block the right nostril with the thumb and exhale and inhale a breath through your left nostril, then switch. Block the left nostril with the ring finger and exhale and inhale a breath through the right nostril.

Practice alternate-nostril breathing in this way for ten or twenty minutes in the morning and again in the evening, and do it about ten times throughout the day for two or more minutes each time. You can breathe according to whatever rhythm or pace you find comfortable. You can use your heartbeats to measure the count. Slow is always good.

You can also incorporate box breathing into the practice of alternate-nostril breathing: exhale 4, hold 4, inhale 4, hold 4. Another traditional prana yogic rhythm is exhale 4, hold 2, inhale 4, hold 2.

Day Twelve: Breathing and the Four Dimensions of Awareness

Today, we bring together the mind and breath in a creative way. Consider that there are four dimensions of awareness—that is, your awareness can be internal or external, and it can be narrow or broad.

You can focus your awareness on one point in your body, or you can spread your awareness out to every cell in your body. You can focus your awareness on a single external object in your environment, or you can expand your awareness to include everything around you.

Today we take advantage of an ancient Chinese bit of wisdom: "Where attention goes, energy flows." We want to practice consciously sending breath-energy into the four dimensions of awareness. Use your imagination, use visualization. Use deliberate, willful intention to direct your breath into these four dimensions.

Start by focusing on a point a couple of inches below your navel and in the center of your body at that level. This point is called the *dan tien* or *hara*, the center of gravity in the body. Breathe into that place. Spend a few minutes focused on sending every breath to that place. You could focus on a joint or an organ or some place in you that needs healing or strength.

After some time, switch dimensions. Focus your awareness on your surroundings, or let your awareness shift to your entire body from head to toe. Send breath to every cell in your body. After a while, focus on some specific external point or object: a flower, a tree, the second hand on a clock, or some sound in the distance. Send your awareness and your breath-energy out to it like a laser.

You can even combine dimensions: focus on your whole body while looking at or listening to something or someone. This comes in handy if you want to track your internal reactions to the words or actions of another. Try it when you are caught up in the news of the day on TV. As you are watching the program, focus on the feelings in your body.

There is a story about Galileo: When he was fourteen years old, he was in a church, and he began to focus on a chandelier that was swinging in the wind (external narrow awareness). And then he did something that very few people would think to do: he began to count his heartbeats (internal narrow focus). In doing that, he discovered the mathematical law in physics that controls the pendulum: a testament to the power of combining dimensions of awareness.

Who or what controls or directs your attention and your energy? Fear? Pain? Habits? Other people? Advertisers? Miscellaneous impulses and random urges? Using the breath to gather and focus your energy and awareness is a life skill that has benefits beyond measure.

Day Thirteen: Combining Thought and Breath

Choose a powerful word or a phrase, an affirmation or a declaration, and begin to repeat it to yourself with each breath, as if you are literally breathing those words into your being.

Is there a quality or a talent that you want to embody? Is there something that you need to remember or want to remind yourself of? Perhaps you have a power statement, or you are committed to changing some negative or limiting self-talk or internal dialogue. Use the breath to impress your body and mind with a liberating or nurturing thought, affirmation, or declaration.

Equally important as the words or phrases you use are the feelings that come with them, that are created by them. If you follow a thought, it will lead you to a feeling; if you follow a feeling, it will lead you to a thought. This practice is about combining thought and breath to generate beautiful, powerful feelings.

You may recall the words that Ram Dass spoke that day: "The power of God is within me; the grace of God surrounds me." Maybe you prefer the classic affirmation, "Every day in every way, I am getting better and better." One of the most powerful affirmations I was ever given was "I am always already free!" Breathe that one for a while. With each breath, stress one of the words in the statement. Breathe in each word until it percolates down through your subconscious mind to the core of your being.

Maybe you can choose one of the archetypal affirmations taught by Binnie Dansby in chapter 3, such as "I am an innocent child of a gentle universe", or SEAL commander Mark Divine's favorite: "Looking good, feeling good, ought to be in Hollywood!"

What do you value? Freedom? Courage? Compassion? Peace? Clarity? Harmony? Health? Love? Persistence? Patience? Create a power statement, an affirmation, or a declaration, and then put the power of the breath into it in order to create a real and powerful experience of it.

Heartfelt words powered by the breath can transform your mind and your life. Today is a great day to be alive, a great day to breathe new life into your mind and body!

Day Fourteen: Energetic Rapport and Connecting Through the Breath

Today, I invite you to use your breath to express how you feel and to use your breathing to connect to those you love and serve. Breathing is a behavior. In the same way that you can give and receive information with posture, facial expression, and the tone of voice, you can also express yourself and sense others through and with your breathing.

Most of the energy that is transmitted through the breath bypasses the conscious mind and goes directly to the most ancient part of our brain, our gut, our heart, and our soul.

If you want to make someone nervous or put them on edge, just start breathing as if you are getting ready to explode or charge at them! If you want to send a subtle signal of safety, give yourself a long, smooth inhale and a gentle, relaxing sigh of relief through your nose. Put yourself at ease with the breath and others will naturally feel more comfortable and at ease in your presence.

Many expressions, like "Aahhh," "Oooh," "Wow," and "Hmmmm" can be enhanced by consciously adding breath to these vocal expressions and interjections. Mirroring someone's breath can add to your sense of connection and strengthen rapport, in the same way that mirroring someone's posture and demeanor does.

Taking in a long, conscious inhale while nodding in agreement, for example, will give you a deeper sense of the energy under or behind the other person's words, and the other person will have a deeper sense of being heard and understood.

You can use the breath to signal the completion of an exchange; it can give everyone involved a sense that what was just communicated outwardly was thoroughly integrated, agreed to, or accepted internally. You will note that this often happens naturally, unconsciously—for example, at the end of a meeting, just before everyone closes their notebooks and prepares to get up or go on to other things.

We are communicating with our breath whether we are aware of it or not. The idea today is to make those natural breathing responses more conscious and deliberate and to creatively engage in them on purpose at key moments and during social interactions.

We have an ancient, reptilian brain that is hardwired to respond to breathing signals, and if you are a helper, a healer, or in a position of leadership, you can creatively breathe in ways that empower yourself and others.

Pregnant pauses in a presentation can be very powerful, and even more so if filled with a conscious breath or a deliberate and obvious pause in breathing. Plus, some things are often better left unsaid, so today can be a day when you replace verbal outbursts that tend to inflame, escalate, or exacerbate a situation with gentle, quiet, conscious breaths.

For your practice sessions today, chose an emotion, state of mind, or quality that you want to communicate and invent a breath that expresses it. Imagine you are a Shakespearean actor and your part in the play is to dramatically convey a feeling or a message using no words—only breath.

You owe it to yourself to develop a wide repertoire of healthy breathing responses that will help you to really feel, release, and integrate things. Today, engage in Conscious Breathing responses for fun, for greater impact, or to deepen your connection or rapport with yourself and others. Your focus today is to be very creative with your breath and to use it to deepen your connection to others.

Day Fifteen: Charging the Heart

Today, we get right to the heart of spiritual breathing, but first let me say that spiritual breathing need not have anything to do with any religious belief. Many religious people are far from spiritual in the way they live, and many people who are genuinely spiritual have no religious affiliation whatsoever.

Today we want to use the breath to connect with our heart, to open our heart, to be in our heart, and to breathe from our heart.

There are a lot of romantic ideas associated with the heart. We often think of the heart as needing to be protected, as fragile or easily "broken," when in fact it is the most powerful part of us. When we talk about the heart here, we are referring to the pump that circulates blood through the body, but we also mean something much more. "Heart" can refer to the warrior spirit as well as to natural love and compassion.

The physical heart generates an extremely large electromagnetic field. The electrical field of the heart is about sixty times greater than that of the brain, and the magnetic field is about five thousand times stronger than that of the brain. This electromagnetic field can be measured from several feet away.

Through the heart, we can connect with ourselves and others in ways that defy logic and understanding. Through the heart, we can connect with something greater than ourselves, something beyond what the body can sense and the mind can determine from experience.

Consciousness is not a function of the brain, it is a combination of body intelligence and mind intelligence. It seems that the heart is the mediator between the two and a perfect channel for this information and intelligence. It is said that the longest journey we ever need to make is the twelve inches from our head to our heart. Let's dedicate this day to making that journey! The practice is simple: get out of your head and get into your heart. You can even put your hands over your heart as you breathe into that area.

Add to this practice by generating feelings associated with the heart, such as love, compassion, or gratitude. Gratitude may be the highest-frequency, most healing emotion there is. Think of something that makes you feel grateful, or generate the feeling of gratitude for no reason whatsoever. Put yourself into this feeling while consciously breathing into your heart.

Pretty simple, right? But oh so powerful! Start your day with ten minutes of this practice. Stop ten times during the day to breathe gratitude for two minutes, and then end your day with another ten minutes of grateful breathing.

Make your inhales longer, slower, and deeper or bigger than usual, as if you are using your breath to create space inside of yourself—a sense of spaciousness. You can add visualization to the meditation: imagine your heart as a flower opening. This practice of projecting love is not just some woo-woo, New Age hippie thing. Soldiers actually employ it on the battlefield as a way of making themselves more available to intuitive information.

Being conscious of your heart space and breathing into your heart, deliberately generating feelings of love and compassion, appreciation, and gratitude, is a profoundly powerful spiritual practice. Not only does it help you get through difficult times, you will find that your presence affects other people in a very tangible and positive way.

To be conscious is to be spiritual, to be spiritual is to be conscious. When you bring loving consciousness to anything, it becomes a spiritual experience. To breathe into your heart is a spiritual activity, a spiritual experience. I cannot tell you how many times people who were fervently antireligious have reported to me that they had their first genuine experiences of spirituality as a result of breathing consciously into their hearts.

Day Sixteen: Tantric Breathing

Tantra is an ancient path to spiritual awakening, spiritual purification, self-realization, and ultimate liberation.

There are many taboos around sex, yet if it were not for people surrendering to their sexuality—and even celebrating it—none of us would be here. Sexual energy is life energy, creative energy, healing energy, breath energy. Inhibiting or suppressing any one of these inhibits and suppresses all the others; there is no way to block one without blocking the others. A great spiritual teacher once said that "sex is just as sacred as Samadhi." He said, "The bottom rung of a ladder is just as much a part of that ladder as the top rung."

Here are several exercises you can play with today:

In a very sensual way, imagine drawing energy up from your feet to the top of your head with the inhale, and then sending the energy from the top of your head back down to your feet with the exhale. Keep sweeping the energy from your feet up to your head and your head down to your feet as you inhale and exhale. When you get the hang of it, expand beyond the body and begin drawing energy from the center of the earth through you and up into the heavens with the inhale, then draw energy from the heavens down through your body to the center of the earth.

Another meditation is to imagine totally emptying yourself out into everything and everyone in the cosmos with each exhale, and then filling yourself with everything and everyone in the cosmos with each inhale—becoming totally empty and totally full, holding nothing back and leaving nothing out.

Try this: Create a wheel of energy between your genitals and your heart, and circulate that energy with your breath. Draw energy up from your sexual center into your heart and then back around and down from your heart into your sexual center.

Plug this practice into your training protocol today. You don't need a partner to practice tantra; life, nature, existence, the universe, or your own being can be your beloved. (Besides, running off ten times a day for two minutes with your partner might raise some eyebrows!) You can do this meditation sitting at your desk or on the subway. Don't be surprised if people sense something wonderful, special, or radiant about you.

If you do have a partner, give yourself lots of time to practice this:

Facing your partner, either lie down beside each other or sit in chairs facing each other. Simply look into each other's eyes and imagine circulating energy between your partner and yourself.

One partner inhales love energy in through the sexual center and exhales it out through the heart. The other partner inhales love energy in through the heart center and exhales it out through the sexual center. Breathe in the same rhythm as your partner: as you inhale, your partner exhales, and as you exhale, your partner inhales. Welcome to the world of sacred sex, the world of tantra.

Day Seventeen: De-Reflexive Breathing

De-Reflexive Breathing, or Krishna's kriya yoga, is a very beautiful and ancient spiritual breathing exercise and meditation. Until recently, it was only passed on in a strict, traditional way and only to the most deserving and devoted aspirants. But a few years ago it was made available to everyone through the Internet.

Here's the basic method: while physically inhaling, mentally exhale, and while physically exhaling, mentally inhale. Imagine light coming into you as you exhale and light going out of you as you inhale: air and light traveling the same path at the same time, but in opposite directions.

The goal or purpose of the practice is to reprogram or decondition an inherited primal program known as "body identification."

Let me explain it briefly: when a dog sniffs, with the inflow of breath comes the inflow of information. When a dog barks, with the outflow of breath goes the outflow of information. The dog's consciousness is bound to its breath.

Likewise, from birth, when I inhale, my experience is that the breath is coming into "me," and when I exhale, my experience is that the breath is going out of "me." My consciousness is bound to the breath by an inherited survival reflex. This sense of "me" is known as "body identification"—and yet we know that we are not our bodies.

We may have a philosophical or intellectual understanding of this truth—that we are something more, something else, something beyond; that we have a spiritual nature or essence that is greater than the body—and yet we live our lives as if we are our bodies.

Everything in the universe has consciousness, and when we become too fixated on our own separate, individual consciousness, we get out of balance with the rest of the universe, and in a way, we disconnect ourselves from the rest of existence. Spiritual enlightenment or liberation means choosing to expand our consciousness beyond this reflexive body identification and shifting to an expanded awareness of ourselves as something more. We identify with a higher self, or what has been called our true nature.

When we were small children, growing and learning about the world, we needed a sense of a separate self in order to keep our bodies safe. We had to learn the difference between "my body/me" and everything else in the physical universe. If we lived in unity consciousness then, experiencing ourselves as being at one with everything and everyone, we'd get run over by a truck! This primal reflex that gives us a separate sense of self is a useful survival program and a convenient social device. It need not be destroyed or denied. But we do need to soften it, and to awaken to a more expanded sense of ourselves. War and violence, scarcity and lack are extensions or projections of this inherited belief in separation: "It's us or them!"

Normal breathing keeps this inherited reflex alive and active in us, and De reflexive breathing is meant to neutralize it. De reflexive Breathing frees us from a survival program that has outlived its usefulness. It is time to really understand that to be against anyone or anything is to be against ourselves or a part of ourselves.

Don't worry, you won't forget to duck if a rock is flying toward your head. You will not lose your ability to survive in the physical world. In fact, when you embody your higher self you become safer and more secure than ever.

Try this meditation now: when inhaling, imagine light pouring out of you. When exhaling, imagine light pouring into you. You are mentally inhaling as you physically exhale, and you are mentally exhaling as you physically inhale.

It might help you to think *out, out, out* as you inhale and *in, in, in* as you exhale. You can also use your hands to represent the light, drawing your hands toward your face as you exhale, and moving your hands away from your face as you inhale.

I hope you get this. It may sound complicated, but it is actually quite simple. Reread it a few times and practice it as you do.

Day Eighteen: Zen Breathing

One of the central tenets in Zen is "beginner's mind." This is the ability to look at what is as it is, in the present moment, without projecting anything from your mind or your past onto reality. Conscious Breathing is a perfect way to bring yourself totally into the present-moment reality.

The archer has always been a symbol in Zen, so we are going to use archery as a metaphor for our practice today. You see, the same dynamics involved in shooting a bow and arrow also apply to breathing. Both archery and breathwork involve combining powerful physical forces and sharp mental focus.

When the archer draws the bowstring back, that is the inhale. When the archer releases the bowstring, that is the exhale. There is that special moment when mental focus and physical power come together: the target is clearly in view and everything is lined up perfectly. In that moment, there is nothing to do except let go and let the arrow fly.

The arrow is your intention. Generate a heartfelt intention as you breathe in, and then when you breathe out, release the intention along with your exhale. In this practice, you are the archer, you are the bow, you are the arrow, and you are the bull's-eye.

As you inhale, your breathing muscles are stretching and building up physical force. As you generate an intention, you are building up mental force. When your lungs are full, there is nothing to do but let go. The air will release by itself. You don't need to push, you don't need to force, you don't need to blow: you only need to let go.

Today, you want to get familiar with that natural breathing reflex and put it to work for you. When the inhale is full, you don't need to blow or push or force the air out. All you need to do is let go and relax, and the exhale will happen by itself.

Is there a goal or an outcome you wish to achieve or see manifested in reality? Focus on your intention while you inhale, and then simply let go, relax, and let the reflexive power of the exhale set that intention into motion for you. Maybe you have a wish or a prayer, or perhaps you desire to support someone somewhere with your loving intention. Use your breath to do that.

Inhale and generate a heartfelt intention; exhale and release that intention out into the world and into your life. Let the natural power of the breath be the force behind your intention. Each time you inhale, generate the intention as if for the first time. Each time you exhale, relax and let the intention go as if for the first time.

In this way, every breath can be a prayer and a blessing. Your arrows can be things you need to release. Your arrows can be negative thoughts and emotions. Your arrows can be a past trauma, a fear, a doubt, a resentment, or anything you no longer need or want to hold on to. Your arrows can also be positive; they can be arrows of love, peace, and joy.

The Saint Francis Prayer comes to mind: "Lord, make me an instrument of your peace. Where there is hatred, let me sow love; where there is injury, pardon; where there is doubt, faith; where there is despair, hope; where there is darkness, light; where there is sadness, joy."[18]

Day Nineteen: Fountain Breath

Imagine sitting or standing in a pool of water or light. Draw that liquid light up through your body to the top of your head with the inhale; then release the breath out the top of your head and let that light shower down around you like a fountain, returning to the pool.

Keep circulating the energy like this with each breath. You can also allow the energy to pour through your arms and out your fingertips as well.

Allow the energy to clean and purify and brighten your being, allow it to pour out into the world freely.

You can also imagine your body like a flower or a tree: the breath rising up through the stem or the trunk and exploding out the top, blossoms at the end of every branch, releasing a glorious, divine fragrance.

Or you can keep it simple: a fountain of breath rising up through the body and flowing out the top of your head, showering down energy all around, again and again.

Adding a feeling of love and gratitude, generating feelings of peace and compassion, or visualizing your favorite color of light can bring this breathing meditation to life.

Day Twenty: Relaxed Subtle Energy Breathing

This practice involves breathing in a very imperceptible way, so that from the outside it appears that you are not breathing at all, but on the inside the experience is very big and very rich. You are breathing pure energy, and the air moves in and out in a very subtle way. The focus is on silence, stillness, spaciousness, and very subtle breathing. Most people are good at sitting still and being quiet, at least on the surface. But very often, they are like ducks: cool and calm on the outside, but paddling like heck underneath. Today we want to create inner stillness, inner peace, and a deep, quiet spaciousness while breathing in the most subtle, almost imperceptible way we can.

Putting your hand under your nose, you will barely feel the air moving in and out of your body. To do this practice you need to be very relaxed, quiet, and still, with no demands on your time or your energy. It may feel like your breath is just hovering in some neutral place—yet you experience moving or "breathing" energy in and out consciously.

In fact, you *are* barely breathing. The focus is on deep stillness.

At the same time, you want to create a sense of open spaciousness that is within you as much as around you. The focus is on subtle energy breathing with no sense of boundaries or borders. This energy is indeed in and around everything and everyone. It is not personal; it is universal, and you are consciously moving and directing it.

Day Twenty-One: Rebirthing Breathwork

I have saved what I feel is the best practice for last. This is by far one of the most powerful breathing practices on the planet today. The pattern is quite simple: active inhale and passive exhale, with no pauses or gaps between the breaths. You are breathing in a continuous, connected, circular rhythm. Breathe into your heart, and remember that you are not just breathing air, you are breathing energy. That is the Rebirthing Breathwork technique in a nutshell.

Consciously pull in the inhale in a gentle, active way, and then release the exhale without the slightest pause. Snap the exhale loose, set the exhale free; release it quickly and completely—don't blow, don't push. Don't control the exhale at all. As soon as the exhale is over, start the next inhale right away without a pause.

One way of experiencing this practice is: you pull the inhale in and keep pulling, actively producing an extra stretch or expansion of the inhale. Then, when you stop inhaling, the exhale simply happens by itself. You "do" the inhale; you don't "do" the exhale. It is a reflex; it just happens by itself when you stop pulling in. We learned this on Day Five. We called it "engaging the exhale."

The Rebirthing Breathwork technique means that the breathing is continuous. The inhale connects seamlessly to the exhale, and the exhale merges with the next inhale; the inhale turns into the exhale, and the exhale blends into the next inhale.

Active inhale, passive exhale. Consciously pull the breath in and expand; deliberately release the breath, relax, and let go. Breathe in and out through the same channel: breathe in and out the nose, or in and out the mouth, but don't breathe in the nose and out the mouth.

If ten is full and zero is empty, then you want to touch eight and three with every inhale and every exhale. And remember, you are breathing energy, not just air.

You want to get the breath up high into your chest and feel those spaces expand and relax. That does not mean you are blocking the breath from flowing to the abdomen. Keep your belly relaxed and that will happen naturally. Just make sure to focus on breathing into the chest, into your heart space. Feel it stretch and release, expand and relax.

Your breathing needs to be active and full enough to trigger an energy experience, and you need to be relaxing completely on every exhale. Try to stay relaxed even as you inhale in an active and powerful way—that is, don't use any unnecessary effort or produce any tension on the inhale. It's a skill: full, powerful, yet gentle and relaxed inhales.

After a few minutes you should start to feel energy sensations: buzzing, tingling, vibrations, electrical sensations. Open to them. Breathe and relax into them. Remember that all your body's feelings are safe. Your feelings cannot hurt you. It is safe to feel your own energy.

If the energy becomes too intense, ease off on the breathing, but don't stop. Keep a gentle wheel of breath turning: active inhale, passive exhale. Make your breathing softer, gentler, not so deep or full; but make sure to keep your breath moving in a connected rhythm, to keep the energy moving and flowing until everything clears, releases, integrates, or subsides on its own.

Throughout the process, physical sensations will come and go, as will thoughts, images, memories, and emotions. In fact, the emotions can be very deep and seemingly endless. People often experience infancy patterns or re-experience and release childhood traumas. The idea is to breathe and relax into, through, and out the other end of whatever arises in your consciousness. Trust your process. Nothing will come up that you cannot breathe through.

Let whatever wants to happen in your body happen. Welcome whatever presents itself. Give attention and space to whatever happens, and don't try to control or manage anything. Stay focused on simply keeping the breath moving and relaxing with every exhale.

• • •

Rebirthing Breathwork is an advanced technique that I mentioned earlier that is best practiced with a good guide or coach. It is possible that you can trigger a process that will continue for an hour or more, so be prepared! One idea is to start by mastering the technique called "Twenty Connected Breaths." It was created by Leonard D. Orr, the founder of Rebirthing Breathwork.

Do the conscious, connected breathing as described: active inhale and passive exhale, with no pauses or gaps between breaths. But just do a set of twenty breaths to start, and make every fifth breath a big, cleansing breath. That means you do four short, quick, connected breaths and then one big, long one; four short breaths and one big one; four short, one long; four short, one long: twenty breaths all together, all of them connected.

Do a set of twenty connected breaths right now. Before you start, get a sense of your energy. Practice internal awareness. Do a set of twenty connected breaths and then observe your internal state again. Notice how you feel before and after the exercise. You can do several sets of twenty connected breaths, or you can let your practice morph from the outset. For example, you might take ten or fifteen short, connected breaths and then two or three big, long, cleansing breaths, then another set of ten or fifteen breaths without a pause and another two or three big, long, expansive inhales and sighs of relief. Rebirthing Breathwork is also called "intuitive-energy breathing," so you can follow your intuition.

Experiment with speed, volume, and intensity. Remember the rules: active inhale, passive exhale, no pauses or gaps between the breaths. Inhale and exhale merge into a continuous, circular, connected breathing rhythm. Breathe in and out the nose, or in and out the mouth, but don't breathe in the nose and out the mouth.

Got it? Then go for it! Awaken your electric body. Activate your energy body, and let this energy do its work on you and in you. This breathing can produce a deep, transformational experience. Trust life. Trust the energy. Trust your process. Trust your body. Meet and greet whatever arises with your breath. If you feel the need to stop, don't stop, just adjust your breathing—make it slower or quicker or more subtle, but keep breathing, no matter what!

As I mentioned earlier, this process is one that is best done with a coach or facilitator. For a list of qualified breathworkers, or to find out if there is a certified Rebirther near you, contact office@breath mastery.com.

AFTERWORD

The results we get from practicing breathwork depend on what we put into it. And I'll say it one more time, the most important thing we need to put into breathing is awareness—conscious awareness. When we open and relax into the energy in the breath, when our breathing is coordinated, and the breathing mechanism is strong and flexible, when we add the secret sauce of conscious intention to the breathing, then you have at your disposal something that can help you to accomplish and achieve anything.

Play with the breathing exercises, techniques, and meditations you have learned here. Experiment with and explore this handbook as much as you need, coming back to it for information and inspiration.

If you want to reach the highest levels of mastery, then focus on and practice relentlessly the two basic aspects of breathwork: Breath Awareness and Conscious Breathing. Remember to get into the habit of observing your breath and taking control of it whenever you can. Remember too that the ultimate key to experiencing all the promised benefits is turning your daily practice into a natural way of being.

The way we approach breathwork reflects the way we approach life. By observing your breathing, you can learn a lot about yourself. You gain the wisdom and ability to gently follow your intuitive flow, to know when to take charge of the breathing, how to harness its power, and when it's time to get out of the way and let the breath breathe you.

There are four stages of learning any skill. We start with "unconscious incompetence." For example, let's say you know nothing about pianos; you don't even know they exist. You are unconscious of pianos and of course incompetent when it comes to playing one.

Just knowing that a piano exists isn't enough. In fact, when you sit down at a piano, you quickly realize that you probably are at a loss to do anything with it. And that is the second stage of learning any skill: "conscious incompetence." Now you know that you have an instrument at your disposal, but you have yet to discover, explore, and develop all the ways that you can use and enjoy it. My job and the purpose of this book is to take you to the next level, and that is "conscious competence." I am here to wake you up to the fact that your breath is an amazing instrument that you can use to create an extraordinary life.

If you practice the exercises and techniques described in this book, you will become consciously competent at breathwork. But this third stage is similar to having to think about how to sit, how to position your hands, and where to put your fingers moment to moment when playing the piano. Maybe you can play a few simple songs, but you can't really make music. To do that you must reach the fourth stage of learning: "unconscious competence."

This level of mastery can be reached with the help and support of a good coach, but it really depends on one thing: deep practice. This means discipline and dedication. Fortunately, breathwork delivers immediate results. The practices are fun and enjoyable, the benefits tangible and real, so it's not at all a chore. I am one of the laziest people I know, so if breathwork demanded anything like hard work, if it wasn't easy, I'd be the last one to do it!

Leonard Orr once said: "Most religions make getting to heaven so hard that even God couldn't make it!" We call spiritual breathing "grease for the slide home!" I am a big believer in the simple things, the basic things in life. It seems to me that the simplest things, the most basic things are always the most powerful. And what could be more simple or basic than breathing?

I hope by now you know that you have, right under your nose, an amazingly versatile tool and an unbelievably powerful force at your disposal. And that you are now ready to bring the practice of breathwork into your everyday life, to prove to yourself that you have the same abilities as the great masters, saints, yogis, mystics, healers, and warriors of ancient and modern times. Peak performance, optimal health, and ultimate potential are now within your reach.

I'll end with two affirmations that I invite people to consider and accept before a breathing session. The first is: "Something I believed would be very difficult, complicated, and take a long time, can actually be quite simple and easy, and can happen very quickly." (Feel free to formulate this into your own words.) This belief is important, because we all naturally assume that if we have a grand goal or desire, it will be difficult, be complicated, and take a long time and a lot of work to achieve. Neutralizing or reversing that deep belief can create a space for miracles.

The second is: "No matter what was true about me yesterday, today anything is possible. No matter who or how I am today, tomorrow I can be anyone, any way. No matter what was true about me in the last moment, right here, right now, in this moment anything is possible." (Again, put this affirmation into your own words, and let it sink deeply into your subconscious.) When we look at our limitations, we tend to think: *That's just how I am.* I am here to say that you can be any way you choose. And if you are willing to change, then the breath will be right there to help you make that change.

I want to thank you for reading this book and taking this journey with me. I hope you will actually practice, because the proof is in the pudding. The breath is the closest thing I have found to a magic wand, but what we get from the practice depends on what we put into it. The best thing we can put into it is passion and enthusiasm and a bit of time every day to practice. One of the things I have learned is that when we are feeling angry, it is because we are generating the energy of anger. When we experience sadness or fear, it is because we are generating the energy of sadness and fear. We create our experience of reality in life. And if you are ready to create love and peace and joy and inner freedom, or excellence in any field, then the breath is ready and waiting to serve you.

We are going to finish this journey by starting a new one. Some-one—I think it was Bob Mandel, one of the original rebirthing breathworkers—said, "Completion is a great place to start." Let's fin-ish by starting today, right now!

ACKNOWLEDGMENTS

I would like to thank Hedda Leonardi, my student and friend, for being the spark that got me to sit down to write and bring this book into being, and for supporting and encouraging me throughout the process.

I also want to thank Emily Han for helping me turn a mountain of articles and stories, seminar transcripts, and training materials into something more organized and understandable. Thanks to Zhena Muzyka for putting Emily on my case, and for sensing the importance of breathwork in her own life and deciding that it was time to bring breathwork to the world in a bigger way. Thank you to Haley, Alexandre, Amy, Yona, and the entire team of talented professionals at Simon & Schuster, Enliven Books, and Atria.

Thank you to everyone who contributed to my work and to this book: Ela Manga, Mark Divine, Stig Severinsen, Wim Hof, James Cook, Leonard Orr, Binnie Dansby, Luba Bogdanova, Michael White, Linda Heller, Peter Litchfield, Pat Gerbarg, and so many others—too many to list here. Thank you to Rugile and Debra, and to my office, admin, and technical teams. Thank you to all my teachers and students and associates, and to all of my seminar organizers, hosts, and sponsors, Thank you for giving me the opportunity to do what I love.

Special thank you to Louise, who has supported me in everything I have ever done. Without her, I would never have finished this book, and to Gulnur for allowing me to follow my heart and to live my dream. And thank you to my sons, Danny and Dennis, and everyone in my family, for giving me the time and space to do my inner work, and for always being there when I need a place to hide out, to take a break, or just feel normal for a while!

Thank you to my parents, Pauline and Joshua, for giving me the freedom and safety and unconditional love I needed to learn and grow at my own pace, and for allowing and even encouraging me to break family, social, and even religious rules in order to find my own way in life.

Last, I thank the breath itself for being the life in me, and myself for sticking to this path through thick and thin over all these years, and for knowing that the best is yet to come!

ADDITIONAL RESOURCES

www.breathmastery.com
www.danbrule.com

Check out our weekly blog and subscribe to our monthly newsletter and Breath & Breathing Report. Get information about seminars and workshops, and find an affiliated coach or trainer near you, or become one! Join the Breathmastery Inner Circle to access a huge and growing collection of books, articles, reports, seminar notes, workshop handouts, audio/video recordings and transcripts: training materials going back more than forty years!

Instagram @danbruleofficial
Twitter @danbrule
Facebook.com/DanBruleBreathmastery
LinkedIn.com: Dan Brulé—danbrule1008@gmail.com
www.BreathTechApp.com

As a training companion to this book, I invite you to download *Breath Tech*, the new breathing app. Enjoy audio and video lessons and instructions on nearly one hundred breathing exercises, techniques, and meditations. Choose one of Eight Paths based on your breathwork goals, and plan your self-paced Breath Mastery Training.

Track your progress as you advance from Student, to Apprentice, to Specialist, to Expert, to Master.

www.o2collective.com/breath-mastery-fundamentals

The *Breath Mastery Fundamentals Course*. Includes twenty-five video modules, plus a training manual with charts, and a private Facebook chatroom/forum.

www.TheBreathingFestival.com

The largest gathering of Breathwork teachers, trainers, researchers, students, and enthusiasts in the world!

www.bajabiosana.com

The Breath Mastery Training Center in Los Cabos, MX, and venue for the Annual Breathmastery Retreat and Immersion Intensive.

www.breathmastery.ru

The official home of Dan Brulé and Breath Mastery in Russia.

ENDNOTES

1. Richard P. Brown, MD and Patricia Gerbarg MD, *The Healing Power of the Breath: Simple Techniques to Reduce Stress and Anxiety, Enhance Concentration, and Balance Your Emotions* (Boston, MA: Shambala Publications, 2012).

2. Stephen W. Porges, PhD, "The Polyvagal Theory: New Insights Into Adaptive Reactions of the Autonomic Nervous System," Cleveland Clinic Journal of Medicine, 76 Suppl 2, S86-90, 2009: http://www.ncbi.nlm.nih.gov/pmc/articles/PMC3108032/.

3. Dr. Patricia Gerbarg, personal communication to author, July 11, 2016.

4. Richard P. Brown, MD, Patricia L. Gerbarg, MD, and Fred Muench, PhD, "Breathing Practices for Treatment of Psychiatric and Stress-Related Medical Conditions," *The Psychiatric Clinics of North America* 36(1): 121-40, 2013: https://www.researchgate.net/publication/236089528_Breathing_Practices_for_Treatment_of_Psychiatric_and_Stress-Related_Medical_Conditions.

5. Richard P. Brown, MD and Patricia Gerbarg MD, *The Healing Power of the Breath: Simple Techniques to Reduce Stress and Anxiety, Enhance Concentration, and Balance Your Emotions* (Boston, MA: Shambala Publications, 2012).

6. David O'Hare, *Heart coherence 365: A Guide to Long Lasting Heart Coherence* (France: Thierry Souccar Publishing, 2014), Kindle, 301-304. Translated from the French by Michelle Hallworth.

7. "Wild Geese" by Mary Oliver. Accessed August 21, 2016. http://www.rjgeib.com/thoughts/geese/geese.html.

8. Stanislav Grof and Christina Grof, *Holotropic Breathwork: A New Approach to Self-Exploration and Therapy* (Albany, NY: State University of New York Press, 2010).

9. Dr. Ela Magna, "My Energy Codes" (unpublished manuscript, 2016), PDF file.

10. Mark Divine, *8 Weeks to SEALFIT: A Navy SEAL's Guide to Unconventional Training for Physical and Mental Toughness* (New York: St. Martin's Griffin, 2014).

11. Barnet Bain, *The Book of Doing and Being: Rediscovering Creativity in Life, Love and Work* (New York: Atria Books, 2015).

12. Paramahansa Yogananda, *The Autobiography of a Yogi* (Los Angeles, CA: Self-Realization Fellowship, 1998).

13. Foundation for Inner Peace, *A Course in Miracles* (Tiburon, CA: Foundation for Inner Peace, 2008).

14. Leonard Orr, *Breaking the Death Habit: The Science of Everlasting Life* (Berkeley, CA: Frog Books, 1998).

15. Dr. Michael Ryce, *Why Is This Happening to Me, Again? And What You Can Do About It!* (Theodosia, MO: Dr. Michael Ryce, 1996).

16. Michael Hewitt-Gleeson, *Software for Your Brain, 3rd edition* (Victoria, Australia: Wrightbooks, 1997).

17. Gurucharan Singh Khalsa and Yogi Bhajan, *Breathwalk: Breathing Your Way to a Revitalized Body, Mind, and Spirit* (New York: Broadway Books, 2000).

18. The Saint Francis Prayer. "Catholic Online." Accessed August 21, 2016. www.catholic.org/prayers/prayer.php?p=134.

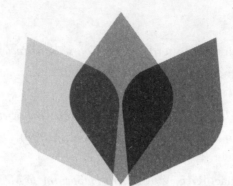

ENLIVEN™

About Our Books: We are the world's first holistic publisher for mission-driven authors. We curate, create, collaborate on, and commission sophisticated, fresh titles and voices to enhance your spiritual development, success, and wellness pursuits.

About Our Vision: Our authors are the voice of empowerment, creativity, and spirituality in the twenty-first century. You, our readers, are brilliant seekers of adventure, unexpected stories, and tools to transform yourselves and your world. Together, we are change-makers on a mission to increase literacy, uplift humanity, ignite genius, and create reasons to gather around books. We think of ourselves as instigators of soulful exchange.

Enliven Books is a new imprint from social entrepreneur and publisher Zhena Muzyka, author of *Life by the Cup*.

To explore our list of books and learn about fresh new voices in the realm of Mind-Body-Spirit, please visit us at

EnlivenBooks.com | **f/EnlivenBooks**